JUBILEE NURSE

Jubilee Nurse

Voluntary District Nursing in Ireland, 1890–1974

Elizabeth Prendergast and Helen Sheridan

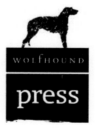

WOLFHOUND

press

Wolfhound Press
33 Fitzwilliam Place
Dublin 2
Tel: +353 1 485 3749
Fax: +353 1 676 6580
Email: info@wolfhoundgroup.com
www.wolfhoundgroup.com

ISBN: 978-0-86327-980-5
ePub ISBN: 978-0-86327-983-6
Kindle ISBN: 978-0-86327-984-3

A catalogue record for this book is available from the British Library.

Printed in Ireland by Colorman Ltd.

Contents

Acknowledgements

Elizabeth and Helen would like to thank, for their years of patience and generosity, their husbands David and Brendan and all of their daughters. Tess O'Leary of Wolfhound Press deserves a special merit for her patience with the production of this book.

The authors have been astonished by the thoughtfulness and interest of people all over Ireland who have helped in a variety of ways to make the research and publication of *Jubilee Nurse* possible. They especially wish to thank all those interviewed for their hospitality and kindness. It was a great privilege to meet with two exceptional women, Mary Duffy and Mary Nolan. The authors express their deepest sympathy to both families on their recent loss.

The extensive research for this book was made possible by the assistance and encouragement of the people listed below in no particular order:

Brian Donnelly, National Archives, Bishop Street, Dublin
Mary Larkin, a friend, indeed, of Birr Castle, County Offaly
Kathy Purcell of Airfield Trust, Dundrum, Dublin 14
Liam Kenny, Broadfield, Naas, County Kildare
Helen McNutt, Donegal County Archives, Lifford, County Donegal
Joseph H. McGrath, son-in-law of Mrs Doolan
Mathew Bradby, Christine Widdowson and Rosemary Cook of the Queen's Institute, London
Fergus Flynn of the Department of Health, Hawkins House, Hawkins Street, Dublin 2
Pieta Taaffe and Elizabeth Ryder of the Queen's Institute for District Nursing in Ireland
Authors and historians Margaret Ó hÓgartaigh, Catherine McCann, Therese Meehan and Dr Muiris Houston have been of invaluable support. The authors are very grateful to Lord and Lady Rosse for allowing them to view the collection of private papers relating to the district nursing association in Birr. They were gathered by Anne, the

Countess of Rosse, and chronicle almost 70 years of dedication and, in her words, 'value, not patronage'.

Several people have helped in a variety of ways and will know themselves why they deserve mention in *Jubilee Nurse*. They include Kieran Corrigan of Wolfhound Press, Jenny Bulbulia, Michael Fewer, Gail Wolfe and Lisa Hyde.

In keeping with a strong theme throughout this book – that thank you is a less valued currency now than it was in the period covered by the study – the authors do appreciate all the encouragement and assistance they received from so very many people in this long venture. Thank you!

Introduction

The development of a district nursing service in Ireland is rooted in the work of thousands of individuals who dedicated their time and energy, often on a voluntary basis, to improving the standards of domiciliary healthcare for those who truly needed it. This invaluable contribution to Irish society has unfortunately been overlooked by historians. The people who provided such an important service to those in need for almost a century have largely been forgotten. The object of this book is to open a much-needed discussion on this matter and to grant some recognition to the aforementioned individuals for their quiet and tireless efforts.

The Queen's Institute of District Nursing, a branch of the Queen Victoria Jubilee Institute for District Nursing in the United Kingdom, was established in Ireland in the late nineteenth century to train hospital nurses in the skills required for providing care to the 'sick poor' in their own homes. Upon completion of training, the Queen's Institute dispatched these nurses to districts throughout Ireland. Responsibility for the supervision, payment and wellbeing of each nurse fell to district nursing associations affiliated to the Queen's Institute which were present in every town and village to which a nurse was sent. These associations were run by a voluntary committee, usually made up of wealthy and well-respected members of the local community, and duties ranged from initial application to the Queen's Institute for a nurse, to fundraising efforts to cover her costs and the provision of support to the nurse – financial, social and emotional. The immense contribution of time, energy and money by this committee, and members of the local population generally, cannot be exaggerated. These individuals would welcome the nurse into their community and their homes and offer her employment and respect. In return, each nurse worked long and unforgiving hours caring for her neighbours, their infant children and elderly relatives. Many nurses dedicated their entire

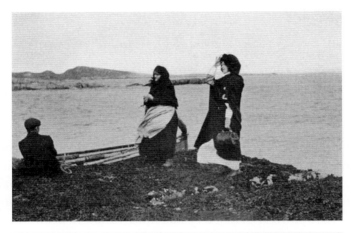

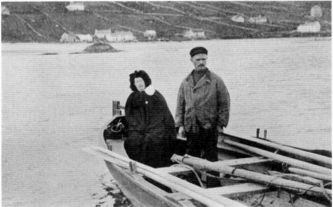

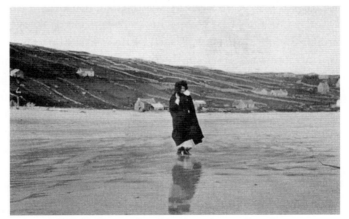

Nurse MacMahon being taken to Aranmore Island, Donegal, 1904.
Courtesy of the National Library of Ireland.

adult lives to the district, remaining in one area from completion of training until retirement or death.

The first chapter, 'Queen's Nurse' offers an overview of the professional and personal lifestyle of the nurses themselves. It examines the reasons these women chose this profession and the factors which led to their selection by the Queen's Institute. It describes the education of the nurses, the relationships they maintained with their superiors, patients and co-workers, and their living conditions.

The Queen's Institute was meticulous in the records it kept, from which much of the information herewith was sourced, and operated with extreme efficiency and cost-effectiveness. The second chapter, 'The Queen's Institute' details the foundation of the Queen's Institute in England and shortly thereafter in Ireland. This governing body, like many of the committees we meet in this book, had male representatives but was dominated by hard-working and committed women. The proficient day to day operation of the Queen's Institute was due in no small part to the fact that the women who supervised it were, for the most part, Queen's Nurses themselves. They understood the needs of the nurses, and were sympathetic to them, but were also acutely aware that for their continued employment they had to have great reserves of tact and resilience.

Although each nurse was paid a modest salary, the committees of district nursing associations affiliated to the Queen's Institute operated on an entirely voluntary basis and the cost of a nurse was primarily covered by fundraising efforts within the local community. This began a tradition throughout Ireland of charity and the organisation of events and community occasions in order to raise money for a worthy cause. Fundraising in itself is something which, when done right, can secure significant returns. It does, however, require precise coordination and great creativity. Throughout *Jubilee Nurse*, the voluntary efforts of the district nursing associations, the Queen's Institute and their local populations are chronicled, offering an insight into the remarkable organisational skills of this network of individuals and groups, and reflecting the generous and unwavering efforts offered by those involved in the provision of this domiciliary care service. Greater examination of their work would be a valuable resource to those involved in fundraising today, whatever the cause, as it offers an example of a highly successful and innovative model for its time which could effectively be applied today.

The third chapter examines the operation of these district nursing associations and their committees, their daily management and vast fundraising efforts mentioned above. A full list of the district nursing associations affiliated with the Queen's Institute throughout Ireland can be found at Appendix I, including dates of affiliation and closure and the number of nurses associated with each district. This list also notes the names of certain nurses who held particularly lengthy positions within their districts and deserve remembrance for this reason. The fourth chapter of *Jubilee Nurse* presents profiles of several district nursing associations and a number of Queen's nurses. This information has come from various sources, including the original records of the Queen's Institute and first-hand interviews with former nurses.

Lady Rachel Dudley was the wife of the viceroy of Ireland when she set up the Lady Dudley Scheme for the Establishment of Nurses in the Poorest Parts of Ireland in 1903. Lady Dudley's Scheme provided nurses to parts of the country, usually along the western seaboard, where the local population did not have the financial ability to support a nurse through local fundraising. The salary of each Lady Dudley's nurse was paid from a central fund in Dublin and her employment, home and transport were administered by Lady Dudley's committee. The scheme, which, in reality, took the form of one large district nursing association, particularly in its interactions with the Queen's Institute, is examined in the fifth chapter of this book, in addition to the work of Lady Aberdeen and the Women's National Health Association (WNHA). During the early evolution of the voluntary district nursing service studied in *Jubilee Nurse*, the WNHA led the way. As with the Lady Dudley's Scheme, the WNHA was established by the wife of a viceroy, Lady Ishbel Aberdeen, in 1907. Its primary function was to educate the population on the prevention of the spread of tuberculosis. Many of the committees which formed these women's associations in the first decade of the twentieth century developed into district nursing associations that continued to employ a Jubilee nurse until the 1970s.

This examination of viceregal patronage of the district nursing scheme is followed by a short chapter of case studies. These first-hand accounts of nurses' treatment of patients, which have been extracted predominantly from the annual reports of the Lady Dudley's Scheme, illuminate the difficulties and joys the nurses encountered. It shows both the varied and repetitive elements of their work and also affords an opportunity for us to meet some of their patients, the official records of whom were mostly destroyed to preserve their confidentiality.

The authors were first introduced to the subject of the Queen's Institute and its nurses when Elizabeth Prendergast, in her research of a separate matter, uncovered a large box of files at the archive of Airfield House in Dundrum, County Dublin, the former home of the Overend family. The box contained detailed reports and correspondence relating to the coordination of Dundrum District Nursing Association between 1898 and 1967. This discovery sparked a consuming fascination in unearthing as much information as possible on the subject in order to uncover the full story of the 'Jubilee nurses'. The authors were rewarded with an immeasurable amount of primary material – annual reports; correspondence; medical records; accounts ledgers – gleaned from archives, libraries and private collections throughout Ireland and the UK, and previously studied in very little detail, if at all. The most valuable source of information in researching *Jubilee Nurse*, however, was the interviews which the authors conducted with former nurses and their families, neighbours and patients. These personal memories and anecdotes served to fill in any gaps in the research and portrayed a valuable, vital and often charming representation of the lives of many of these women.

The title of *Jubilee Nurse* is one which refers to the name colloquially assigned to these women. Although technically titled 'Queen's nurses', district nurses who were dispatched by the Queen's Institute were often sent to districts throughout rural Ireland at a time when popular opinion of Great Britain and, in particular, the crown was one of distrust and animosity. The automatic association with the monarchy generated by the nurses' official title was very unfortunate as the majority of these nurses were young Irish women with no particularly unionist beliefs and the ethos of the

Queen's Institute generally was one of non-sectarian treatment for all those in need, regardless of social background, religion or political belief.

The only agenda behind the work of the Queen's Institute, its district nursing associations and their Jubilee nurses was the improvement of the standard of living of their patients, at a time when such a standard was set to a very low threshold across the country. They did this by educating communities, offering valuable advice and, most importantly, by leading by example. Throughout a very turbulent period of Irish political and social history, they offered a stable and supportive presence to communities. The Jubilee nurses discreetly continued their daily work without any great fanfare and, in turn, their accomplishments went virtually unnoticed. Perhaps this is because of the aforementioned association with the British crown; perhaps it is because they were women. Or perhaps it was simply because they did not demand any significant recognition but preferred to carry out work which they saw as simply necessary and which, in the words of one Jubilee nurse, 'had to be done and there was nobody else to do it but yourself'. Whatever the reason that the story of the Jubilee nurses has been so overlooked until now, it is hoped that this book will offer some well-deserved acknowledgement of the work of all involved in the provision of domiciliary care under the supervision of the Queen's Institute in Ireland.

District Nursing Associations Affiliated with the Queen's Institute of District Nursing

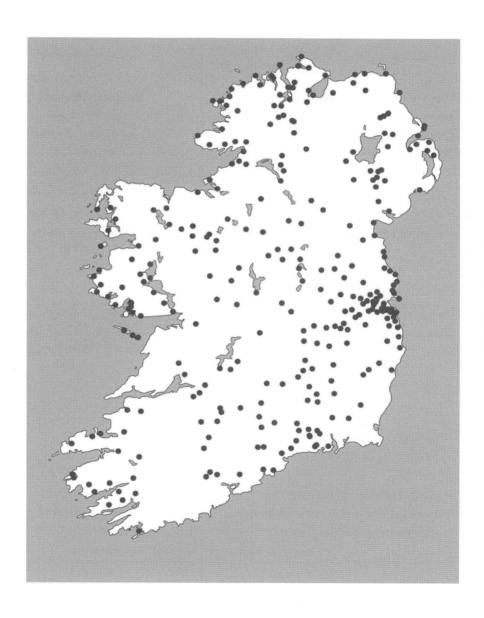

Structure of the Voluntary District Nursing Scheme in Ireland

Queen's Institute of District Nursing

Established in Ireland in 1891
Ceased training in 1968

Known at various times as:
Queen Victoria's Jubilee Institute of Nurses
Queen's Nursing Institute
Queen's Institute

Responsible for:
Training
Supervision
Inspection

Training Homes in Dublin
St Patrick's Protestant Nurses Training Home
1876–1968
St Laurence's Catholic Nurses Training Home
1892–1953

District Nursing Associations	**Lady Dudley's Scheme**
1891–1968	1903–1974
Operated in over 320 towns throughout Ireland.	Maintained 49 nurses across the Western Seaboard.
Each district nursing association supervised and maintained its own nurse.	All nurses under Lady Dudley's Scheme were maintained from a central Dublin office, akin to one large district nursing association.

CHAPTER 1

Queen's Nurse

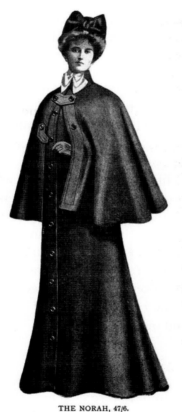

DEBENHAM AND **FREEBODY**

CONTRACTORS TO THE
PRINCIPAL
LONDON HOSPITALS
AND
MANUFACTURERS
OF THE

QUEEN'S
JUBILEE
NURSES'
UNIFORMS.

NURSES' CLOAKS,
NURSES' UNIFORMS,
NURSES' BONNETS,
NURSES' CAPS,
NURSES' APRONS,
and Complete Nursing
Equipments.

Detailed and Illustrated Catalogue
post free.

THE NORAH, 47/6.
Cloak as sketch made in showerproof materials, summer and winter weight.

DEBENHAM and **FREEBODY,**
WIGMORE STREET, LONDON, W.

Courtesy of Queen's Nursing Institute, London.

1

Dressed in a pale blue frock with white starched cuffs and collar, in which the silver Queen's badge sat neatly under the chin, and a white apron that was pinned up in front while working, the Queen's nurses wore a dark blue, heavy wool outer cape which later modernised into a gabardine coat. The hat changed little because it was essential to be able to pull it right down over the ears, to stop it blowing away in the wind while cycling the endless roads all over Ireland. They wore laced-up black shoes and carried a large leather bag.

This chapter will not differentiate between Lady Dudley's nurses and Jubilee nurses; they were all qualified as Queen's nurses. Their education, uniform, the regulations they worked by and their home lives were, in reality, highly similar. The only major difference between the working circumstances of these women was that Lady Dudley's nurses were guaranteed to live in a rural district and they did not have the support of a district nursing association (DNA) committee. All of these women were motivated by a similar passion to improve the welfare of the people in their districts. The cliché that nursing is a vocation was, for most of these women, very true.

A description of the working life of a Queen's nurse would be incomplete without first-hand accounts from the nurses themselves. For this reason, reference is made throughout this chapter to individual nurses with whom the authors have spoken in relation to their careers. They offer an invaluable, and often charming, insight into the daily lives of the nurses and represent a far more personable and effective source of information than written records alone. A more detailed description of the career of each of the nurses mentioned can be found at the end of this chapter.

QUALITIES OF A QUEEN'S NURSE

The attributes of a good Queen's nurse were deliberated by many during the establishment of the Queen's Institute for District Nursing. Annie Michie, superintendent for the Irish branch of the Queen's Institute from 1913 to 1926, said at a talk in 1920 that 'the district nurse should have sound health, both in body and mind, have received a liberal education, be possessed of plenty of common sense, resource and tact, a sense of humour, thoroughly interested in and have sympathy with the poor'.[1]

For the organisation, high standards were vital and the bestowing of a uniform and badge to a qualified nurse was a serious matter. Sir Edward Coey Bigger, MD, said of Lady Dudley and Jubilee nurses that 'The nurses of both these organisations are well selected and specially trained for the duties they have to perform. By their skill and devotion they have won the respect, esteem and affection of the poor in every district of Ireland to which they have been appointed.'[2] The nurse's comportment reflected that of the whole organisation, from the institute itself to the committees locally. The work required great stamina. Contact with dangerous contractible disease, without any form of immunisation, was certain. The nurses were required to be on call 24 hours a day, regardless of the weather, and usually on a bicycle covering many miles. Resilience, adaptability and independence were vital as many districts were isolated, and even those that were not involved many weeks of little contact with peers, colleagues or friends. Visiting sick people, pregnant women and infant babies in their own homes required great tact and empathy.

The most important quality required of the nurse, however, was that she wanted to do the job and that she enjoyed the social interaction in order to become a vital and respected part of her community. Former Jubilee nurses, and those who remembered them, support this idea that enjoyment of the job was essential. Mary Duffy, a Jubilee nurse for the Taughboyne district in Donegal from 1945 until her marriage in 1951, and many others, have remarked that they loved being a community nurse because they were aware that the work they did had the potential to make a real difference to many lives. Jubilee nurses were part of a community health system that was not fully evolved, and many bridged the gap which potentially formed between the work of social workers, home help and psychologists. Maura Kilmartin, a Jubilee nurse for the Dundrum district from 1952, was married to a local school principal. This relationship gave both professionals a deeper insight into the difficulties of many children in the district.[3] Many of the longstanding nurses developed unique characteristics and eccentricities that enabled them to survive and, in many cases, to elicit valuable support and assistance from the members of their adopted communities.

For the Queen's Institute, the task of ensuring an intake of women for training from the 'right' sort of background to fulfil the requirements on the many diverse types of districts was a great one. It is probably not necessary to mention that there were no male Jubilee nurses and none were sought. Much discussion in the early years centred on whether it was appropriate to employ 'ladies' or women of a more lowly status as some of the work involved dispatch into horrific slums that may have injured the sensibilities of 'gentle-women'.

In 1896 the superintendent for St Patrick's nursing home made her views clear:

> It should be borne in mind that it is far more difficult to procure suitable nurses for district work than for any other branch of the profession. This arises from the high attainments necessary for a district nurse. In addition to her full training in hospital work, she must be a good woman, as well as a clever nurse. Sympathy, ability, energy, tact, and judgement must be combined with good health and unusual powers of endurance. It has been our experience that among educated gentle-women only can we find those who are able to exercise authority and influence, without hurting the tender susceptibilities of our poor, in their own homes.[4]

Research into the background, religion and previous experience of the nurses was assisted by the level of detail that was recorded in the roll of the Queen's Institute. According to Margaret Damant in an extensive biographical profile of Queen's nurses in Britain between 1910 and 1968, 'they were generally intelligent and spiritually inspired women from a predominantly middle-class background'.[5] Many of the Queen's nurses in Britain were from Ireland. Research in the Irish records shows a strong bias in favour of applicants from farming families. In the early stages some applicants' fathers were referred to as 'gentlemen farmers' but the great majority of women were from rural backgrounds. Some came from middle-class trading families – the daughters of civil servants, teachers or Gardaí (or Royal Irish Constabulary officers). If the candidate did not have any previous experience, 'home duties' were very acceptable.

With the increase in the number of nurses being sent to the west of Ireland for Lady Dudley's Scheme, the ability to converse in Irish was an added bonus although not essential as it was presumed they would pick up the language quite quickly. In 1903, Nurse Hedderman was dispatched to the Aran Islands without a word of Gaelic – 'a stranger in a strange island'.[6] She managed the language difficulties initially with some help from locals who had a little 'Béarla' and eventually acclimatised. According to Mary Quain, a Jubilee nurse located in the Connemara Gaeltacht at Carraroe in County Galway in the late 1930s and who had school-level Irish, her experience was of social isolation in the beginning but she soon acclimatised despite admitting that she was never fully proficient in the native language.[7] By the middle of the twentieth century, many of the locals had relatively good English, even in Gaeltacht areas.

Most women applying to the Queen's Institute were more established in their careers as nurses and, on application, they ranged in age from mid-twenties to mid-thirties with some qualifying in their forties. In order to train as a Jubilee nurse, a woman required previous hospital training and midwifery qualifications. Many had worked as staff nurses in various institutions before beginning their six months in one of the training homes. In the view of the Queen's Institute, the training of a district nurse was about 'how to adapt the knowledge and skill she has gained in hospital to the circumstances of her district patients and how to make the best of the unfavourable conditions and limited appliances available in a poor home'.[8]

Basic hospital training in anatomy and physiology, first aid, asepsis and medication was important. It was reinforced in the training period and the nurse was encouraged to continuously update her skills. It was remarked in the reports of annual inspections of many district nursing associations that nurses may have 'out of date methods'.[9] This was, of course, not unusual when a nurse was in the same district for 20 or 30 years but was still noted by the inspector. Some nurses availed of educational courses in order to update their skills but, for most, the month of holiday leave every year was precious time to be spent with their families rather than embarking on further nursing training. Inspections of the districts were viewed as a chance to update nurses. A pamphlet entitled the

Handbook for Queen's Nurses published in 1924 said: 'Inspection Visits are encouraging, helpful, and stimulating, and the nurse will find herself looking upon the Inspector as a friend who understands and appreciates her difficulties, and who is always ready to help her or her Committee with expert advice and assistance.'[10]

In the early stages of the Queen's Institute in Ireland, many of the women had trained as hospital nurses in England or Scotland. Later nurses were often recruited from local Irish hospitals and were all also qualified as midwives. Annie P. Smithson, a Jubilee nurse from 1901 to 1920 and the author of a number of popular novels based on her real-life experiences as a nurse, describes cutting short her training in a London hospital in 1898 to go to Edinburgh Royal Infirmary, Scotland to train as a Jubilee nurse in order to take up a post as a district nurse in Ireland. Nurse Smithson trained for two years in Edinburgh before being sent to St Patrick's Nurses' Home, St Stephen's Green, Dublin for six months. She did not appreciate being a 'probationer again' but could not be a Queen's nurse until she had passed her examinations and inspections on the district.[11]

The training of a general hospital nurse had changed very little from the Victorian era, during which time it was implemented under the direction of Florence Nightingale, until very recently with the introduction of the university degree in nursing. Prior to this, nurses learnt their profession in a practical manner on the wards, with the support of occasional lectures and exams. The hierarchical structure of hospitals at the time was rigid and disciplined.

Hospital training was described in 1920 by recently qualified Nurse Vera Matheson speaking at a conference on 'The Nurse and the State'. She described the system as dependent on the quality of the trained nurses, ward sisters and matrons to behave with respect towards probationary nurses and trainee nurses and noted this was not always the case. She stated that 'discipline is always necessary in community life, but it is the manner of the discipline that is resented, not its fact'.[12] For many nurses this arbitrary, often verging on despotic, system led them to seek another way to practise their nursing skills. In the narratives of many Jubilee nurses, this desire to seek a less rigid means in which to practise their skills was an important part in the decision to commit to the district nursing service. Mary Quain expressed this to Therese Meehan in an interview: 'Her view after completing training in 1935 was that she loved nursing but not the strictures placed on nurses' practice in hospitals.'[13] Maura Kilmartin had been a staff nurse in the Meath Hospital and had a continuing association with the hospital for many years after she became a Jubilee nurse. She said in an interview that she loved being a Jubilee nurse as there was 'nobody breathing down your neck' and felt that she could achieve a lot because of this independence. Jubilee nurses preferred their autonomy on the district. Control over their duties and the ability to build up permanent relationships with their patients and their families was an important freedom.

Midwifery training was also vital for a Queen's nurse. In the early stages of the Queen's Institute, when dual qualifications were not frequent, some nurses may not have completed midwifery until after they had commenced their work in the district. Nurse Annie P. Smithson provides an example of this practice. She worked in the district of Gilford, County Down before leaving to return and finish her training as a midwife. The Queen's Institute sometimes sponsored general nurses to train as midwives. In 1929, thirteen nurses had their midwifery fees paid.[14] Lady Aberdeen also sent nurses to Edinburgh in 1908 to study as special tuberculosis nurses.[15] Even when all Queen's nurses were fully qualified in domiciliary midwifery it was not always a service that was required in many districts and a nurse would become out of practice. Towards the end of the scheme there was a financial incentive in some districts for the committee of a district nursing association to offer midwifery to patients because of the government grant that was available for this service. If the nurse was out of practice or not willing to provide domiciliary midwifery in her area she would request a transfer and a new nurse would be provided for the area.

TRAINING OF A QUEEN'S NURSE

The training of nurses by the Queen's Institute was carried out in St Patrick's Nurses' Home and St Laurence's Nurses' Home in Dublin and in a separate training home in Derry. St Patrick's Home functioned primarily in the training of Protestant nurses with St Laurence's Home established in 1891 for the training of Catholic women. All nurses' homes were regulated by the Queen's Institute and operated in the same way as very large district nursing associations, providing a domiciliary nursing service to their local communities. They did not function as hospitals with inpatients but effectively acted as residences for staff and trainee nurses to use as a base when visiting patients in the surrounding districts.

The nurses' homes provided accommodation for the six-month training period until 1965. From this date forward, all nurses in Ireland were trained at St Patrick's Nurses' Home but were accommodated in local lodgings. The nurses' homes provided very comfortable living conditions. According to Francis Aylward, superintendent for Ireland, in a lecture in 1954: 'The superintendents are vigilant in making those homes real homes, not institutions, and the nurses when off duty are granted the personal freedom due to educated fully trained professional women.'[16] An anonymous nurse offered a description of St Patrick's Nurses' Home in the *Queen's Nurses' Magazine* in 1905. 'Each nurse has a separate bedroom and

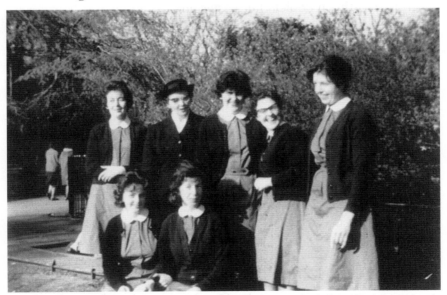

St Patrick's Nurses' Home at St Stephen's Green was a happy place for trained nurses to learn about district nursing and gain practical experience visiting homes in the local area. Phyllis Nelson and Mary Byrne, interviewed for this book, became lifelong friends during their time in St Patrick's. They are pictured here in St Stephen's Green Park in the 1960s with Miss Morgan, their supervisor (with hat), and some other students. Courtesy of Phyllis Nelson.

there is a delightfully restful nurses' sitting room at the back of the house with a well stocked bookcase and a reception or music room with a good piano … It is an old-fashioned house, large and airy, and has been made comfortable and convenient in every way.'[17]

Supervised visits to the districts were conducted in the mornings and formed the fundamental basis of the training experience for the nurses. Each morning the nurses went with a qualified supervisor to the district. Afternoons were occupied by lectures given by renowned Dublin medical specialists. Examinations would follow the tuition received during these lectures in subjects such as fevers, hygiene and gynaecology. The nurses also received a course of cookery lectures and demonstrations.[18] The hours were long and often there was great pressure on the nurses, who received one Sunday off each month, thereby allowing them freedom from Saturday after dinner. 'Those who have friends in Dublin can stay with them. Those who remain in the home breakfast in bed on Sunday morning.'[19]

Annie Smithson depicts her experience as a nurse at St Patrick's Home in her first novel, *Her Irish Heritage*, published in 1918. She evokes a contented, well-organised and supportive environment. Smithson describes meal times as very formal. 'Miss McFarland (matron) enters almost immediately, grace is said, the nurses drop into their places and the meal commences.'[20] The nurses' time was tightly supervised and one of Smithson's heroines, Mary Carmichael, a staff nurse at the fictional St Columba's Home (based on St Patrick's Home) is constantly rushing for meal times. 'Mary Carmichael got through her morning's work and reached St Columba's with just five minutes in which to change from bonnet and cloak to cap and apron and to generally tidy herself up for dinner.'[21]

The morning rounds involved the 'probationers' going with a qualified nurse or supervisor to visit the sick and elderly and was referred to as 'slumming' by the nurses in *Her Irish Heritage*.[22] The areas visited by the trainee district nurses represented some of the poorest parts of Dublin city. Shock at the poverty of the homes they visited in the inner city was a common sentiment among nurses of all periods throughout the history of the training homes. From Victorian times to the early decades of the twentieth century, scarcity of food and hygiene and the consequential bad health was endemic in tenement slums. The Jubilee nurses who trained in the late 1960s still remembered great poverty in all the districts around the centre of Dublin. They all fondly recall, however – despite the poverty – that the kindness and wit of their patients sustained them through their training.[23] Nurses Mary Byrne and Phyllis Sproule, based in St Stephen's Green, remember the endless stairs of the tenements and the lovely people who were delighted to see the nurses coming up from the street.[24] Maura Kilmartin trained in St Laurence's in 1952 and remarked that, even then, the poverty was grim. She gives an example of this poverty in her description of how nurses always brought a shilling to put in the meter so that there would be light or gas to heat water in the flats, at least for the duration of their visit. They always brought their own soap and towel because such supplies were non-existent in the tenements.[25]

Some districts were located quite a significant distance from the nurses' home and were reached on bicycle or public transport such as trams. The nurses were accordingly allowed an unlimited number of tram tickets.[26] In 1904, 2,142 cases were nursed and 36,702 visits were paid by the nurses of St Patrick's Home. The work was distributed as calls were received in the nurses' home from the doctors in the area and referrals were often given from neighbours and family of sick people. This daily inventory then became the day's visits for the nurses. The Jubilee nurses of the later period remembered in interviews going to St Patrick's to do their reports from the day before and then being given the list of patients and addresses to visit the following day. They were not living in the home at the time and it saved them an extra journey to report in.[27]

Great emphasis was placed on the prevention of the spread of infection. Jubilee nurses often had to visit houses where there were infectious diseases and also call to maternity cases or to check on new babies. The organisation of the work day in order to prevent such occurrences was vital. In 1889 the St Patrick's Nurses' Home annual report proudly proclaimed: 'It may be well to add, that since the Home was founded, not a single instance of the spread of infection, through the agency of the nurses, has been reported, or alleged to have occurred.'[28]

Ruth Barrington, in *Health, Medicine and Politics in Ireland*, says that as new areas of the city were developed, no appropriate increase in the dispensary service was provided. 'Dublin dispensary doctors were responsible for the treatment of approximately 6,220 persons each.'[29] The Queen's Institute and her Jubilee nurses quietly slipped into the gap to support the overstretched service in Dublin's inner city. In 1953 fundraising became untenable for St Laurence's Home. Newspaper accounts of its closing in August of that year bemoan the loss of the valuable service of the fifteen nurses in the area. 'The main sufferers will be the poorer sections of the city, who will be losing a real friend in the person of the familiar nurse in the blue cap and cape, who was always at hand when her services were required.'[30]

Nurse Quain's notes, from her time as a probationer in St Laurence's Home in 1937, illustrate the many subjects covered by the trainees. Several lectures were shared with the trainees in St Patrick's Home on the south side of the city. They cover all of the different elements of the district nurse's practice. A lecture entitled 'District Management' included a large section on planning visits according to urgency, infectious cases and any maternity work that may need to be carried out within the time limits of a busy day. Each lecture is recorded by hand in a legible and clear sequence. There was a series of lectures entitled 'Responsibilities of the District Nurse' which began with advice to gain the cooperation of everyone in the district including the doctor and other professionals, patients, families and the district nursing committee. 'The district nurse has a duty toward her own health and should be an example of healthy living.'[31] In a lecture on 'Record Keeping and Statistics' Nurse Quain and her co-students learned of the different grants the district nursing associations were entitled to and the paperwork that was required for government records such as maternity, child welfare and other statistical requirements. Records had to be kept for the nursing association, for the Queen's Institute and for the nurses' own records as a form of protection against legal actions. A series of lectures from Dr Alice Barry covered the subject of tuberculosis, including the disease itself, preventative measures and the treatments used. There was a section on the public health schemes, specifically focused on tuberculosis, that were in effect at the time, which mentions the sanatoria where advanced cases were sent.

The subjects were practical and took into consideration the nature of the places these nurses were to be sent. Studies were focused on issues such as the necessity for good nutrition, clean air, water supplies and sewage and pointed out all of the serious complications that can occur with general neglect in these areas. They covered subjects such as the duties of a health visitor, whose work could be done by the Jubilee nurse and which was paid for by the county council in the form of a grant paid to the DNA. These lectures covered all of the laws governing maternity and child welfare, school nursing practice, notifiable diseases and their times of incubation.[32]

In recent interviews, Nurses Mary Byrne and Phyllis Sproule, both of whom were trainees at St Patrick's, complained of the time wasted by studying the British socio-medical legislation in the 1960s. The Irish branch of the Queen's Institute had separated from its British origins in the 1920s with the declaration of the Irish Free State. Sheila Pim explained in the *Irish Times* in 1966 that they continued to use the British examinations because it 'kept up the high standard of their work through years when no other training was available'.[33] The nurses said that the superintendents were very strict and that daily inspections of the bag and the uniform, in particular the starched apron, should be pristine and pressed meticulously. Both nurses felt the uniform, described above, was outdated by the time they had completed training. They did not pay for it and it was obligatory that they wore it when they took up their post on the districts.[34]

After passing the exams and inspections, each nurse was the subject of an interview with the superintendent. A page in the roll, or register, of Jubilee nurses was set up for each nurse and her career in the Queen's Institute was recorded vigilantly. The title and badge for the Queen's nurse was formally awarded by the institute. Later nurses remember that is was the Protestant Archbishop of Dublin who presented their badges to them in their graduation ceremony.[35]

The final examination must have been reasonably difficult because several nurses were registered but removed from their first district as they failed on quite a few attempts.[36] Comments on each nurse's page of the roll tended to emphasise her kindness, reliability, consideration, capability, practicality and educational qualities. The newly qualified Jubilee nurse was then expected to work for a year in the district to which she was appointed.

After the closure of the Queen's Institute in Ireland in 1968, nurses who had completed the training period as Queen's nurses and who had more than five years' work on the district were automatically registered with An Bord Altranais as public health district nurses. Those with less than three years' experience were brought to Fitzwilliam Square to An Bord Altranais' headquarters to do a course of eight weeks before they were sent back, usually to their own district.[37]

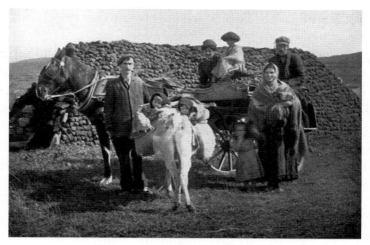

NURSE AND PATIENTS, MALLINMORE, CO. DONEGAL.
Courtesy of the National Library of Ireland.

NURSE AND HER PATIENTS

A handbook for Queen's nurses published in 1924 noted that the conditions of the patients of the district nurse 'vary as much as their surroundings, which may be those of a crowded city or a lonely country area, so she must be able to adapt herself to every circumstance and to deal with every grade of intelligence'.[38]

The importance of overcoming personal prejudices was examined by Annie Smithson in her description of her first district experience between 1901 and 1905. It was an aggressively Protestant area in the North of Ireland and Annie very quickly adopted a very nationalist political view which was supportive of Roman Catholics. She said in her memoirs: 'As individuals, I might not have cared for them, but when a person is a patient, a nurse gives to that person of her very best.'[39]

In her novel *Carmen Cavanagh,* published in 1921, Annie Smithson describes the tension for a young woman in a new district in Donegal.

> She had come amongst these people as their district nurse, she was therefore bound to get to know them intimately; she would share their joys and sorrows, see them under all sorts of conditions – at their best and at their worst. She honestly wished to help them, to be of use to them – one on whom they could depend at all times. And yet she felt some very serious qualms and doubts as to her reception by these people in whose midst she now found herself.[40]

The overriding sentiment identified in our research was the gratitude of patients for the assistance of the nurse. Jubilee nurses were not taken for granted. They were honoured guests in their patients' homes and their arrival was greeted with warmth and appreciation.

The period covered in this study was between 1891 and 1974. Society and the social conditions of people changed enormously in this period of Irish history. The living conditions of the poor visited by district nurses at the beginning of the twentieth century were vastly different from those in place after the social welfare system was secured. To understand the work of the nurse it is necessary to understand the living conditions of the people whom she visited. The work of early Jubilee and Lady Dudley's nurses were, in many respects, similar to aid workers in third world countries today. The philosophy of care was very different from the work done by public health nurses today or even in the later stages of the service. The political context in which the nurses worked was important as it changed how they were perceived by their patients, families and neighbours through the period. Legal, political and medical support for voluntary district nurses changed as it moved from being part of the British civil service to a slowly evolving Irish state health service.

Periods of great stress for communities can be seen in annual reports through the whole study. The First World War, which impacted on Europe between 1914 and 1918, marked an unsettled period during which some of the Queen's nurses were deployed on military service. During the 1916 Easter Rising many of the nurses in both St Patrick's Home and St Laurence's Home tended to those wounded on the streets of Dublin. For several months Miss Annie Michie, superintendent of Irish operations for the Queen's Institute, acted as matron of the Red Cross Hospital at Bray, near Dublin.[41] With the assistance of a grant from the Joint Committee of the Red Cross and the Order of St John, the women of the Hospital Supply Depot made garments and provided the nurses with bales of bandages and surgical dressings throughout this time until 1947 when the grant ceased.[42]

In the early 1920s, when political strife seems to have been our official history, there was a significant food shortage in the west of Ireland due to a few years of bad weather and a failure of crops. The devastating impact of this shortage is rarely raised in discussions of Irish history around this time. In 1921 Lady Dudley's Scheme district of Lissadell was to be closed. 'The committee, at this time of distress and anxiety, when on all sides so many are faced with illness and starvation, earnestly beg for more help to enable them to assist destitute families by keeping the children alive until such time as organised work can be arranged for those members of the family who are able to earn a living.'[43] Their petition failed and the district closed that year. The Lady Dudley Scheme annual report for 1924 describes the monotony of the ceaseless rain. 'The turf is too sodden to burn; and where the inadequate supply of potatoes, small and bad, points to a near state of semi-starvation.'[44]

During the time of the 'Emergency', or Second World War in Europe, there was rationing, increasing prices and the poor were caught in an even deeper poverty trap. Female patients struggled with constant pregnancies, anaemia and hunger. The district nurses were placed at the coalface of this desperation. Mary Quain, in a speech many years later, spoke of her time in the west of Ireland and that 'the outbreak of World War Two had a devastating effect on the people'.[45] Mary Quain was not prone to overstatement. While the work of the nurses was specifically to look after the sick poor of the district, it must have been stressful to have been an intimate, but rather helpless, observer.

Not all districts, however, were rife with poverty. One nurse described being temporarily sent to a suburb of Dublin where she describes visiting rather affluent patients and being brought tea in china service by the maids before going on her way. Caring for family members of the committee was also expected of the Jubilee nurse. Nurse Smithson describes this in her novel *The Marriage of Nurse Harding*. 'Although Nurse Harding's services were primarily intended for the poor of the district, it was an understood thing, that the shop people and others who could afford to pay a subscription to the funds of the association, would be entitled to make use of her services.'[46]

One of the nurses interviewed cared for the husband of the president of the committee of one of the district nursing associations for over a year before his death. While she knew her efforts were appreciated, she was amused that a framed picture of his lordship, as an important member at an influential club, was gifted to her on his passing.[47]

When the Queen's Institute was set up, an essential element of the work was didactic. Teaching people how to prevent the spread of disease was vital and often very difficult because of the deeply ingrained belief in the quacks and customs of the past. Today there is an understanding that some of the folk medicines may have been effective and, if not, they provided harmless assistance in the absence of any other treatment. For early district nurses the use of this folk medicine was a battle that seemed to consume a great deal of their time and energy. Describing dangerous, filthy wound dressings and a horror of the dispensary among the people on the Aran Islands, Nurse Hedderman said: 'Advocates of these customs do not, and will not, give way without a struggle, so that nursing work in the early days was from some points of view a very thankless task.'[48] She was not alone. A Queen's nurse describing district nursing in the west of Ireland in 1904 said that the belief among the people that 'the fairies' or 'the good people' who had caused sickness, particularly that with sudden onset, could not or should not be interfered with was very strong. 'How gently they will reply, and how courteously they will try not to do what you want them to do.'[49]

Hygiene was a large element in this superstition, as the relatives believed that if the sick person was clean and tidy they would resemble a corpse – and this was seen to be bad luck.[50] Florence Nightingale, in her 1881 pamphlet *On Trained Nursing for the Sick Poor*, had insisted that no cures could result without first bringing in fresh air and cleaning the room of the invalid.[51] Her dictums essentially represented the law for nurses for many generations.

In the early years, particularly in the west of Ireland, the greatest problem for nurses was that farm animals and chickens frequently shared the living accommodation with the people. This was described by William L. Micks in his history of the Congested Districts Board.

> Nothing would have enabled a stranger to realise the conditions of home-life as well as visits to the cottages, or in many cases hovels, after nightfall, when there would be found in the same small unventilated structure all the members of the family, with cattle, ponies, pigs and poultry. A stranger would be disgusted and would wonder why the people choose to live in such conditions. It was not a matter of choice.[52]

Through the use of grants, the Congested Districts Board supported Lady Dudley's Scheme by building and repairing suitable cottages for the nurses to live in. Mr Micks said of the scheme: 'The nurses of the Dudley Trust were particularly well trained in their duties; and, apart from actual nursing, they promoted cleanliness and healthy living.'[53]

For the nurse it was essential to prevent the spread of disease, and the importance of clean water and homes and personal hygiene was paramount. In *Carmen Cavanagh*, Annie Smithson describes an outbreak of diphtheria.

> The epidemic had spread so quickly through the villages of Knockbeggan and Carragh that now there was scarcely a cabin without one or two sufferers. Some had the disease slightly, others were as bad as they could possibly be. Sanitation, except in some of the better houses in Carragh, was absolutely nil, and it was a simple impossibility to get the inhabitants to understand the merest elements of hygiene or disinfection. As for isolation – it just could not be done.[54]

While this is a fictional account, Nurse Smithson mentions in her autobiography that Carmen Cavanagh describes her life as a Lady

Dudley's nurse in Glencolmcille, County Donegal from 1910 to 1912.[55] Diphtheria today is almost extinct in industrialised parts of the world due to vaccination, but during its existence in Ireland it had been a very deadly bacterial infection.

While nurses were, of course, not instructed to be condescending, they were expected in the earlier years of the Queen's Institute to have a higher status which the poor would look up to, and try to emulate a refining and educating influence.[56] As living standards and education among the people of the districts improved, the Queen's nurses adapted to the different requirements of the occupation. The authoritarian tone in the nurse's communications with her patients softened. Annie Michie was superintendent of the Queen's Institute of District Nursing in Ireland from 1913 to 1926. In a speech in 1920 for the General Nursing Council of Ireland she reflected this changing philosophy.

> The educational influence of these same nurses is far-reaching, and has done more to raise the standard of living of the poor than any other philanthropic agencies put together. The principal reason for this is that they go to the homes of the poor as working women to help their working sisters, and to show them how to manage with things they actually have in their homes, and not as 'Lady Bountifuls' to give doles in money or kind.[57]

Mary Quain discussed this educational element of her relationship with the people of Carraroe, County Galway in the 1930s with Therese Meehan, lecturer in the School of Nursing and Midwifery, University College Dublin. 'Health teaching and emotional advice were constant themes in Mary's work.'[58] Nurse Quain believed in taking a cup of tea and allowing the people to open up to discussion that allowed them to unburden themselves and, in so doing, help them. She said: 'You could go through an awful lot of work with a cup of tea under certain circumstances.'[59] This philosophy of explaining basic medical information, such as cross-infection, first aid and the encouragement of a healthy diet, in a gentle and friendly manner in the patient's own home was very effective. Later nurses commented that they could smell the tea boiling before the front door was opened and that there was no hope of refusing it.[60]

Being a good educator had another logical rationale for nurses. It was important to teach a family member, neighbour or any other carer how to continue treatments for the patient in the absence of the nurse. The Jubilee nurse always had large districts with many calls on her attention, and even the most ill patients could not monopolise her whole day. On occasion, nurses from Lady Dudley's Scheme wrote letters to the secretary at the head office, chronicling their experiences. Many of these were detailed in the annual reports.

One nurse described the following in 1907: 'A baby with bronchitis, who lived three miles out. I made and put on poultices, and showed the mother how to continue carrying out the doctor's directions until my next visit.'[61] Because of this necessity to transmit orders clearly, the educational objectives of the Queen's Institute continued into the 1950s and 1960s. During her service as superintendent for Ireland, Nurse Quain, and her board, were responsible for policies taught in the training home. The nurses were examined in St Patrick's Home based on their ability to instruct the clients they visited on the district. Qualification reports frequently mentioned the nurse's ability to teach. Generally they were competent to educate people but occasional shyness or other problems made them less effective. In such cases it was hoped they would improve with time and experience.[62] Follow-up inspections some time after dispatch to their new districts were certain and these difficulties, or otherwise, would be mentioned in the subsequent report.[63]

In later years the work of the Queen's nurse often became more that of social worker and social activist. Filling the gaps in the undeveloped health system was a natural progression for the woman who was already well established in the community and who was universally respected and trusted.

NURSE AND HER COMMITTEE

In an article in the *Irish Times* in 1955 entitled 'A District Nurse's Day', Sheila Pim gave an account of a fictional nurse's view of her committee. 'The committee has its uses; some of its members help at the baby club. Some provide linen or can get comforts patients need, some even give the nurse flowers for herself, but mostly they worry about money.'[64] For many years, Sheila Pim was the treasurer for Dundrum District Nursing Association in Dublin. She was also an active member of the council of the Queen's Institute. The subtitle of the article was 'Work, Work, Work', demonstrating the great respect Miss Pim had for the Jubilee nurse. If committee members felt that a nurse was exhausting herself, they ensured that adequate rest was taken.[65]

Voluntary district nurses received very little support from the Queen's Institute except in the form of the annual and sometimes bi-annual inspections. The general belief was that the local committee was there to support the nurse in everyday difficulties. For many nurses the committee members may have been the only people that the nurse was comfortable to socialise with outside of work. The formation of lasting friendships would have been a natural consequence for women working together for years with the same objectives in mind. Nurse Smithson noted in her first district that the honorary secretary, the school mistress, 'won her heart at once'. In a letter to the authors of this volume, Professor James Muldowney, whose mother was a member and passionate supporter of the committee of a district nursing association in Kilkenny, mentioned the lifelong friendships that his mother developed with many Jubilee nurses and fellow committee members during her involvement with the Queen's Institute. Many of these friendships began the moment the new, and often nervous, young Jubilee nurse was met off the train at her new district by a member of the committee.

Queen's nurses met their committees regularly at monthly meetings and whenever there were any administrative jobs to be done with regard to dispensaries, halls or other properties which required management. District nursing association committees were aware that they were not allowed to involve themselves with patients or their families but were conscious of the work the nurse was carrying out through the monthly reports. They met at all the events organised in the community, many of them as fundraisers for the association. In small villages, indeed, there was little chance of *not* meeting the nurse out and about on a daily basis and of having a casual chat. In the case of Lady Dudley nurses, a member of the committee was allocated to liaise with all the nurses in the county she lived in. As the contact of a committee was not available to the Lady Dudley's nurses, social support was provided by the doctor and his family, religious leaders, local teachers and others who were not dependent on the nurse's care exclusively.

The efforts of the nurse were not reflected in the salary she received and each committee was usually aware of this. An interview with Nurse Maura Kilmartin supports this. She mentions the wonderful committee that she was represented by in Dundrum district and the mutual respect among most of its members. Upon her marriage, Maura Kilmartin was presented at the Dundrum district hall with a very generous gift of a tea chest full of good Arklow tableware. It is her belief that the committee made a request to the Queen's Institute on her behalf that she not be retired upon marriage and was therefore able to continue as a temporary nurse following her marriage. When the Dundrum district nursing association closed down, a second gift of £50 was presented to Maura Kilmartin and her colleague nurse. At the time, this represented an extremely generous offering.

However, relationships between the nurses and their committees were not always smooth. Annie P. Smithson frequently admits to having little tolerance for certain committee members. 'All through my nursing career, I consider that these lay committees are the greatest drawbacks to the work of the jubilee nurse. I speak, needless to remark, entirely from the point of view of the nurse.'[66] In April 1917 Nurse Smithson was sent to the Dundrum district in Dublin – which was at the time still a small town and not the large suburb it is today – to a 'loyalist' committee. The Queen's Institute implemented very strict rules that dictated that nurses should remain apolitical and non-religious in their relationship with the populace. Nurse Smithson remembers 1918 as the year she published her novel *Her Irish Heritage*, which was based on the 1916 Rising, and of the elections in which she canvassed in search of independence for Ireland from the British. When, in June 1919, Nurse Smithson hung the Sinn Féin flag from the window of the nurse's house, this proved the final straw for the committee, which already deeply disapproved of her canvassing. Having created a very hostile atmosphere, Nurse Smithson followed the advice of a friend and concluded that it would be better to resign.[67] The Queen's Institute inspector noted on that occasion that Nurse Smithson was a 'capable conscientious nurse unselfish and devoted to her patients. Thoroughly educational in her methods − not always very wise with regard to political matters.'[68]

Although the committee of the Dundrum District Nursing Association never actually dismissed Nurse Smithson, she describes an extremely unpleasant committee in her 1921 novel *Carmen Cavanagh*. The passage, albeit with changed names, was a thinly disguised description of the place and people of the committee in Dundrum.[69] It was not a flattering portrayal.

Nurse Smithson was not alone in having strong political emotions and differences with her committee. Normally the Queen's Institute sided strongly with the nurse in moments of disagreement and it was in the interest of each of the district nursing associations to keep their nurse comfortable. North Coole in County Westmeath appeared to present an exception to this during another political controversy which it witnessed. North Coole's first (and only) nurse was described throughout most of her short-lived career at that district as conscientious, kind, strong and energetic by the relevant annual reports. She left, however, in 1919 because it seems 'she got mixed up with extreme political people and was reported to have neglected poor people who were not of her way of thinking', according to the report on her record in the Queen's Roll.[70] Her sudden retirement was officially attributed to 'ill health'.[71]

Several nurses also felt that some of the ladies on the committees could be rather overbearing and appeared to believe that the nurse was some form of higher servant that they could command. Towards the end of the scheme many committee members were also quite elderly and perhaps a bit out of touch. This was particularly relevant when fundraising events were being run in the town or village and the nurse would be expected to parade in full starched uniform to assist in the gathering of her salary. Nurse Smithson refers to this in her novel *The Marriage of Nurse Harding* when the heroine of the book, Nora Harding, is invited to a district nursing association fundraising garden fête at the big house. 'Nora had been asked to attend − quite a polite invitation, but that it was really in the form of a royal command, she knew perfectly well. Of course, she was expected to wear uniform, and did so – dark linen frock, white apron, cuffs and collar, neat little bonnet tied with the dinkiest of bows.'[72]

On the other hand, social occasions in small towns, such as the nurse's dance, were the annual events to be enjoyed by all, including the nurse. Nurse Mary Duffy met her husband at the nurses' ball in Taughboyne/Carrigens where she had been recently transferred. She was eventually asked by the committee in nearby Newtown-cunningham, where she had settled down with a family, to take over the district. She had a very good relationship with her committee, which supported her for six years after the Queen's Institute had closed down. Some of the members of her district nursing association were interviewed, and their support for her as a neighbour as well as their respect for her professionalism was noteworthy.[73]

The nurses were paid monthly, often in cash, by a member of the committee. One of the nurses remembered waiting for her salary on Christmas Eve and wondering if the 'Lady' would arrive before the shops were closed. When nurses transferred to the public health system the cheque arrived in the post, which they felt was a much less humiliating practice.[74]

At the end of a long and arduous career for the Lady Dudley's nurses there was always that small travelling clock to look forward to. It was inscribed with the nurse's name and dates of service. The inscribed clock may have been a lovely gesture but it is not likely that Nurse Foley of Caherdaniel, County Kerry would forget that she was in service to Lady Dudley's Scheme from 1931 to 1971.[75]

Nurse and the Queen's Institute

Once qualified and given a post, nurses' contact with the Queen's Institute was usually in their annual, sometimes bi-annual, visit from the inspector, a monthly written report, and requests for holidays and transfers.

As mentioned above, nurses were contracted to remain in their district for one year after completion of training. Part two of the contract or 'Nurse's Agreement', signed by the nurse on qualification, clearly indicates the nature of the relationship with the Queen's Institute.

> The undersigned … agrees to work as a District Nurse wherever the institute may require her services for one year from the date of completion of her district training; to abide by the said regulations; and *readily* and *cheerfully* to obey all the rules of the institute to which she may from time to time be subject.[76] [emphasis added]

While this agreement appears dictatorial, the institute generally tried to be supportive of nurses and their wishes. It also reflects difficulties that the institute encountered when newly trained nurses, who were required by the district nursing associations throughout the country, got married or left for other work, particularly to the public health system, thereby rendering themselves unavailable. It seems a bit harsh that in 1949 farmer's daughter Nora Foley of Lisselton, County Kerry was fined £30 for breaking the agreement. She had to leave Stradbally, County Waterford after three months to go home and nurse her sick mother.[77]

The ability of the Queen's Institute to transfer nurses between district nursing associations quickly and without fuss was praised by Sheila Pim in 1966 when she commented that the new welfare state system was far more cumbersome than that previously offered by the Queen's Institute, which managed to operate without the same 'red tape'.[78]

The Lady Dudley nurses reported to the secretary of Lady Dudley's Scheme. They often called in to the office when they were on holidays in Dublin in order to discuss difficulties or improvements required.

Nurses were appointed to districts on an arbitrary basis when they qualified and some instantly settled in and stayed for many years. Some of the nurses in our study, particularly those who qualified in later life, had a significant influence on the districts they were dispatched to. Mary Byrne said she was not given a choice and was very glad she was sent to Naas, County Kildare and not to Valentia, which at the time was still an island off the Kerry coast with no bridge to the mainland. It was to Valentia that a friend who trained with Mary Byrne was sent.[79] Nurse Smithson describes waiting to be appointed to a district in 1906. She said that she was afraid of being sent back to the North of Ireland as 'the Protestant nurses were nearly all sent to the North'.[80] There was a policy of matching nurses with the religious practice of the majority of the population in the district.

When newly trained and awaiting a permanent post, many nurses were sent on holiday relief or to relieve a sick nurse. Some of these temporary posts became permanent. The very remote Lady Dudley's districts appear to have been the first position for many new Queen's nurses, who tended not to stay very long in these posts. In 1910 Lady Dudley's Scheme annual report noted: 'It is becoming increasingly evident that it is not advisable for nurses to remain in these Western districts for more than three or four years on account of the arduous nature of their duties.'[81] By 1911 the limit was just three years of continuous residence in any district.[82] From the Queen's Institute's point of view this could have been useful because district nursing association committees were often quite demanding and required a nurse with experience. So, after a short while in the west, the nurses were glad to be given a less demanding position even if they did have a fussy committee to contend with.

Not everyone was happy to stay in isolated corners of Ireland. Some erratic decisions on the part of nurses had to be catered for by the institute. Annie P. Smithson describes writing to the superintendent in 1912 to inform her that she could not live in the isolation of Donegal any more. She packed and left with effectively no notice. She said she did not care what it might do for her future career.[83] The institute seems to have been understanding of her difficulties and gave her a placement in the dispensary in Charles Street, in the inner city of Dublin, as a tuberculosis nurse, for which she was very grateful. Leaving a district without notice was not an infrequent occurrence and is recorded periodically in the institute records. In any busy district this must have caused great hardship for those dependent on the nurse and particularly for the dispensary doctor awaiting her replacement.

Many nurses, due to ill health, family or other reasons, requested a move. During the annual inspection the nurse had an opportunity, while out on rounds with the Queen's Institute inspector, to put her case forward for a move to a more suitable district, and if a vacancy occurred, they were considered for the new posting. The Queen's Institute believed that these visits by inspectors would act as a support and comfort to the nurses. In reality, this time spent with the inspectors was frequently stressful and a cause of great anxiety for the nurses. The arrival of the official power from Dublin to view one's work was not an occasion that could be taken lightly. Mary Byrne, who was newly qualified and based in Naas, County Kildare, said that the arrival of what she perceived as a 'scary lady' to inspect her records was viewed with trepidation.[84] Sometimes the inspector stayed for dinner and Maura Kilmartin has commented, of her first years at Dundrum district, that the provision of a good nourishing meal for the inspector acted as an added pressure and was rather more expensive than she could afford at the time.[85] Mary Duffy in Donegal also recalled a visit by the inspector, who went on call with the nurse to check how she was received by the patients. They had an awkward call to make to an elderly man, in dire conditions, in an extremely isolated area. They found themselves walking over bog and field to arrive at a stile in a barbed-wire fence. The old man offered to help the inspector over the stile, remarking to the nurse that 'your mother is getting stiff'. Poor Nurse Duffy had to stop herself from laughing out loud until she was at home alone.[86]

Transfers to another district, and even the request of holidays, generated an enormous stack of paperwork. A tiny sample of this still survives in the National Archives in their Department of Health files. Nurses had to be selected carefully and a new application approved by the local committee, and in later stages the relevant county council had to be informed because of its involvement in funding. When a nurse left her district the small staff in the Queen's Institute faced the colossal task of replacing her.

Nurse and the Local Doctors

The relationship between the doctor and his family, the committee and the Queen's nurse was close and interdependent. Indeed in many cases the doctor or members of his family were on the committee of the local district nursing association. This, for most nurses, was a benefit as they could rely on support from the people that were effectively in the same area of practice. There was a strong co-dependency among both sets of professionals in their work and living situations as many doctors had their surgeries in the clinic which was attached to the nurse's cottage.

The Queen's Institute rules, distributed to all district nursing associations, included a comprehensive list of suggested bye-laws for nurses. Four of these bye-laws relate to nurses and the medical men in the district.[87] The principles therein were also delivered to nurses during training. They emphasised the importance of loyalty to the doctor. The Nurse was forbidden from influencing patients in their choice of doctor. It was stressed during lectures how important it was to follow treatment instructions carefully and never to undermine the doctor's position with patients. Communication with the doctor was vital, but just as important was the recording of these messages and reports on patients' progress. Notes and messages were always to be written, even suggesting a slate, because of the danger inherent in verbal messages. A good communication system between nurse and doctor would have prevented needless visits or ensure that any potential problems were detected early.[88] Midwifery was a large part of the practice for rural and some urban doctors, even when there was a Queen's nurse or dispensary midwife provided. Midwifery nurses had to report all cases to a doctor, who was the person in charge, but usually only called on the doctor for a delivery if it looked like there may be difficulties. A written report was imperative, but also a quick verbal assessment on the delivery would have been conveyed.

The practical side of the relationship is illuminated in Mary Quain's memoir, in which she describes the nurse–doctor relationship for a Lady Dudley's nurse in the west of Ireland in the 1930s.

> Nurse and doctor would sometimes meet on the roads while doing their rounds and always stopped to talk over their patients, particularly any problems or puzzling situations. Some problems could be resolved by talking them through, and for some, each might ask the other to make a visit to the patient and do a separate assessment before talking again. While the doctor gave some instructions for treating patients, he left treatment of many problems to Mary's discretion. She valued greatly the doctor's trust in her professional work and judgement, particularly because it gave a boost to her somewhat shaky professional self-confidence.[89]

The dispensary doctor in Mary Quain's district had four Lady Dudley's districts to cover. His confidence in her was probably a matter of survival. In times of stress and epidemic this relationship was strengthened by mutual sharing of the great workload. Nurses were obliged to report contagious diseases to the doctor as a matter of law from 1947 under the Health Act of that year.

As with most human relationships, that between doctor and nurse could not always be guaranteed to run smoothly. For instance, the Queen's Institute inspector had to mediate between the nurse and doctor in Freshford, County Kilkenny in the 1950s following a disagreement. The nurse was eventually transferred and the doctor was much happier with her replacement.[90] Cappoquin District Nursing Association in County Waterford also had some difficulty with the nurse in the 1950s, whose committee said was 'not working with the dispensary doctor'. As a newly qualified nurse, straight from St Laurence's Home, she stayed less than a year and left for a hospital post in England.[91]

Sometimes, however, the nurse was the only health professional in a district. In 1916 the annual report of Lady Dudley's Scheme justified its demand for funding from its readers because of the war in Europe. 'As the medical men have volunteered from many districts, the nurses are the only persons qualified to render medical aid of any kind, thus the great importance of maintaining the full number becomes apparent.'[92] The number of Lady Dudley's nurses dispersed throughout the west of Ireland that year was 27. Many island communities were without a doctor, especially in times of bad weather, and relied entirely on the nurse for all their medical care. Inisbofin island, as described by Annie Michie in 1920, was '15 miles from the nearest doctor and 7 of them over open Atlantic. [The nurse] has no telephonic or telegraphic communication with the mainland and is often cut off from it for weeks at a time on account of storms.'[93] Inisbofin only got its first Queen's nurse in 1935. It was never properly affiliated as a district.[94] It appears always to have been supplied with a publicly funded district nurse.

But even when there were several doctors within a district, the nurse was the first to be consulted. Maura Kilmartin remembers that every morning in Dundrum in the 1950s and 1960s, she would pray that there would be nothing too serious for her to deal with. The people called to her for everything because they could not afford the doctor unless it was an absolute emergency. She also remarked that there was a different, but no less important, set of relationships with the health board medical officers visiting the schools. After a morning administering vaccinations in a school it was a pleasant break to go to lunch with the doctor. There was also an equally significant relationship with the dentists visiting the schools and rapport would have been important to ensure problem children, and their teeth, were not allowed to slip through the net.

Voluntary district nurses were trained to provide for the sick poor in their own homes and, because of this, they reported principally to the dispensary doctor for the district. The dispensary doctor no longer exists in Ireland. The dispensary system, which was established in 1841, divided the country into dispensary districts, each with a medical officer who was paid a salary from local rates. Patients were seen based on a system of tickets – black for treatment in the dispensary and red for a visit to the patient's home. They were initially distributed by the County Poor Law Guardians.[95] According to Dr Murray of Galway, the doctors knew the poor in the district very well and did not actually require the ticket system. By 1922, the system was administered by the local Home Assistance Officer from the County Board of Health and Public Assistance.[96] Dispensary doctors continued for the duration of our study but the system completely changed to the general medical service in 1972.

Dispensary doctors in the early days, in rural areas in particular, were frontier men who cut a lonely and very strenuous path. The *British Medical Journal* of 27 January 1906 noted the death due to typhus fever of Dr Hickey of Spiddal, County Galway. He was the sixth dispensary doctor to have died in the district in the previous ten-year period.

> Here is a district 65,000 acres, 23 miles long with 6,000 peasants. The salary is £150 and £15 for sanitary duties. The medical officer out of this must provide a horse and car, a house, food and clothes for himself and family. There is no private practice. It certainly is a puzzle why anyone would want the job. Stone breaking would probably be better; it would certainly be less risky.[97]

The lives of dispensary doctors did improve a bit as the years progressed, but these working conditions had started from a very low standard threshold and most still had enormous districts to cover right to the very end. They had very little time off as most districts had only one doctor who was, like the Queen's nurse, on call almost all of the time.

Carrick-on-Suir District Nursing Association, County Tipperary, was in its second year of existence in 1903 when it noted the cooperation of its 'medical men' and that 'it was the general opinion now that we could not do without a nurse in Carrick'.[98] In 1903 the doctor would have dispensed many of the medications that had to be compounded using a pestle and mortar, mixed and put into a suitable method for administration either by oral suspension, poultices or liniments. When the nurse arrived, a lot of this grind fell immediately onto her list of routine tasks. The Queen's nurses were trained to make up their own poultices and ointments for treatment of the many different ailments on their rounds. The nurse did this in her own kitchen probably, at the same time as she was sterilising rags and suitable material for dressings by oven baking or boiling. Much of this gruelling manual work was still being done by Queen's nurses at the end of our study.

An example of a sensible and progressive nurse–doctor relationship was described by Mary Duffy in rural Donegal. She said Dr White arrived shortly after she was sent to an enormous rural district in the county and they worked together in various different areas for 36 years. He was described by some of his patients in Newtowncunningham as a great GP and a good maternity doctor.[99] Mary Duffy worked with other doctors but the dependability of the relationship with Dr White ensured that they had similar opinions on matters. They were able to assist each other greatly with ideas and shared advice each day after daily clinics and school supervisions, over the scones baked by Mary every morning. Then they would head out on their respective visits to the housebound sick. Later, in her second district of Newtowncunningham, Mary went home first to give her children dinner after school.[100] The level of trust and combined knowledge of the people would have ensured that many emergencies never happened, which was a primary goal of a good community care system.

The close relationship between nurse and doctor tipped into the romantic in the case of Annie P. Smithson. This was dreadfully unsuitable as the handsome doctor was already a married man. Annie drew on her experience of the emotions of lost love in several of her novels. In her autobiography she described the progress of the relationship. 'From our first meeting we had been attracted to one another with that irresistible force which attracts as surely as a magnet.'[101] Writing of the inevitability of gossip in a small community, she says: 'In the first place our position as nurse and doctor, which must, of necessity, bring us into close contact, shielded us a good deal; in the second place we were both favourites with our patients.'[102] Annie asked for a transfer and left the district broken-hearted. 'It was all over, those three years of comradeship with the one man whom I had ever really loved.'[103] In her novel *Carmen Cavanagh*, the Lady Dudley's nurse manages to win over her doctor but, instead of living happily ever after, she loses him to an epidemic of diphtheria.[104]

Nurses, whose concern for their patients was paramount, often complained of the doctor who was not so energetic. Some dispensary doctors were, in fact, downright eccentric. Matthew Ganly of Ballinasloe, who lived for many years next door to the local Jubilee nurse Agnes O'Grady, commented in an interview that the people of the district were very dependent on the nurses' quick wittedness as the dispensary doctor was, for many years, well-meaning but not reliable. It was against the rules of the institute for a nurse to influence patients in their choice of doctor. Diplomacy was, once again, a prerequisite for the job.

The district of Naas ran into serious difficulty with a young Dr Murphy in November 1902. He refused to work with the nurse who had been in the district for seven years before his appointment as dispensary doctor for the area. This left the association committee with a problem because if the doctor did not need the nurse, she effectively had no function in the district and neither did the association. The committee was, it seems, in full sympathy with the nurse, 'who might not be the easiest person to get on with' but had never generated complaints before from doctors, committee or subscribers. The doctor claimed his disagreement was for 'purely personal reasons'.[105] Despite efforts by several dignitaries in the community to mediate, the doctor was totally intransigent. The flexibility of the Queen's Institute once more came to the rescue and Nurse Walshe was given a new district. We do not know if there were any more difficulties with the doctor.

NURSE AND THE LOCAL PRIESTS

The Queen's Institute recommended that district nursing associations should enlist the support of the churchmen of all denominations to support their committee. The Jubilee nurse would have been aware of the necessity for a good rapport with all the community leaders in her district. As Irish society became more biased in favour of the Roman Catholic Church through the twentieth century, the parish priest's influence, particularly in the area of voluntary work, was obvious and considerable.

Mrs William O'Brien in her book *My Irish Friends* describes Emily Gillespie, the much-loved Jubilee nurse of Mallow, County Cork from 1901 to 1922, who seemed to win over people of all persuasions. This was through a period of deep political turmoil in Ireland and the new curate, later Bishop of Cloyne, 'became one of nurse's devoted co-workers'.[106] Enlisting the support of the churchmen was easy for a woman who was also caring for those in the crucial stages of their lives.

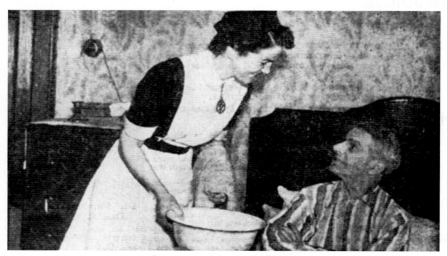

Courtesy of the *Irish Times*.

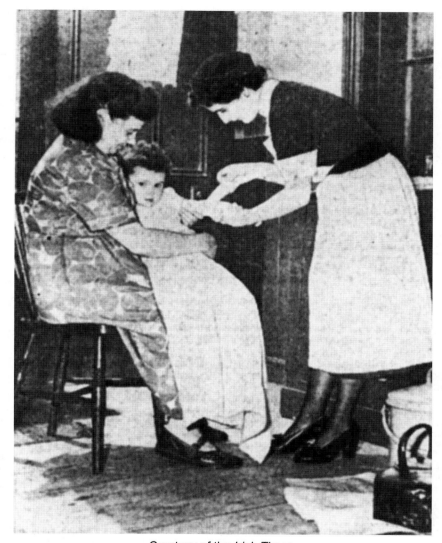

Courtesy of the *Irish Times*.

The Lady Dudley's Scheme was always aware that without the support of the parish priest, or other clergy, fundraising was impossible. In 1917 the aid of the clergy was noted as vital in encouraging patients to contribute to the expenses of the nurse. In May 1965 it was still a matter of discussion that parish priests be sent a letter explaining the expenses of running a district and asking that local collectors be given more support within the communities.[107] Many

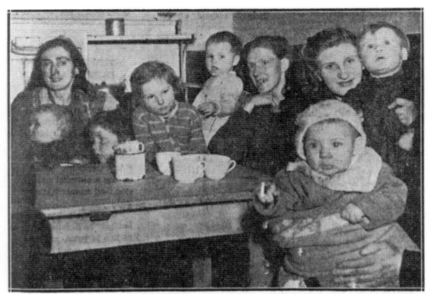

Dundrum and Ballinteer Nursing Association's party in the Dundrum Library, at the re-opening of the baby clinic.

Courtesy of the *Irish Times*.

district nursing associations were set up by these priests once they could see the value of the Jubilee nurse in a community. In the 1940s and 1950s very few district nursing association committees did not include the parish priest or his curate.

Epidemics were unavoidable events and in her novel *Carmen Cavanagh* Annie P. Smithson describes an outbreak of diphtheria which takes the life of the dispensary doctor. She also tells of the heroic behaviour of the parish priest in the community during these times of stress: '... there's nothing special in what he's doing – it's his work and any priest would do the same.'[108] This solidarity with those serving the community in the face of great danger and hardship was a vital part of the support that these professionals provided to each other. The religious faith of patients, in the absence of effective medicines, was a healing aid and can still be a powerful tool in human recovery today. District nurses in tune with their community were aware of how little they could achieve without the support of the confidant of the people. Mary Quain describes a complex relationship with her parish priest in Carraroe, County Galway. She respected his interest in the parishioners but

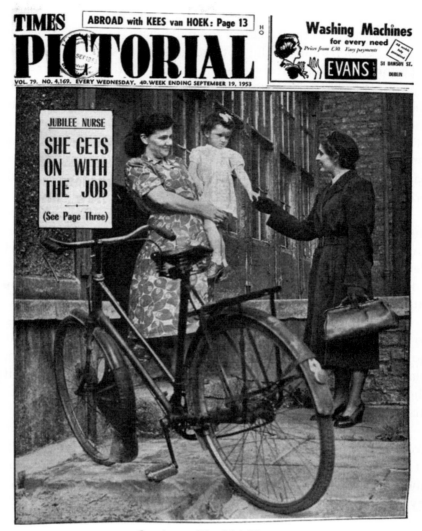

Courtesy of the *Irish Times*.

had to be tactful when following his suggestions regarding her patients and their lives. He was, however, aware of her commitment and respected her abilities.

THE WORK OF THE JUBILEE NURSE

'The work was there to be done and there was no-one but yourself to do it.' This was, according to her colleague and great admirer

Dr Vincent Pippett, the mantra of Mary Kiernan, the last Jubilee nurse to attend to the Wicklow town district.[109]

Most Queen's nurses did not specialise professionally and were therefore intimately involved in every facet of their patients' lives. The duty of care did not apply simply to the individual patient but to the entire family. They delivered and washed the babies and visited them for weeks after their birth, cared for them through epidemics of anything from measles to poliomyelitis, inspected them in school and watched as they grew up as neighbours and grandchildren of patients. They would then deliver the next generation, repeat the process, and wash the dead in preparation for their last journey.

Crucial events in patients' lives did not often happen between the hours of nine and five. When a baby comes into the world, it happens when it does, not when it would be convenient. Similarly, death can be shockingly fast or excruciatingly slow. The Queen's nurse cared for the patient but also offered a calm and professional support for the deceased's family and friends.

One of the nurses we interviewed described getting ready to go to a dance one Sunday night. She was called to the parish priest's house to find the old canon had died. That was the end of her planned evening. She put on her uniform and spent the night with the housekeeper washing and dressing the remains of the old man instead of jiving the night away.[110]

It was not possible for the nurses to dedicate themselves to any area of special interest. However, some districts had a high number of maternity cases and others contained larger elderly populations and it was the luck of the draw if the nurse preferred the majority of the work in the area where she was sent. If she stayed in a district long enough her interests grew and evolved with the population and its changes. No matter how organised the nurses were, no day was the same – around every corner was a new adventure. According to Francis Aylward, the superintendent for Ireland in 1954, at an international conference that year: 'The day's work of each Jubilee Nurse is all absorbing and strenuous but it is never monotonous.'[111] The Queen's Institute inspectors usually went for a day with the nurse to get a feel for the work and the reception they received in the homes of the people. If the Queen's inspector felt there was not enough work in a district to keep a nurse busy, especially in Lady Dudley's districts, it was suggested the district be closed and the nurse transferred.

The act of visiting patients in their own homes was referred to as 'rounds'. This was the essence of the work for a voluntary district nurse – and still is for public health nurses today. Planning the rounds was vital, according to a lecture given to Mary Quain in 1936 at St Laurence's Home. 'The wise district nurse will vary her routine so that the patients realise that there are others to be attended, and that the acutely ill must be seen first.'[112] Mary Quain described a day in the life of a Jubilee nurse in 1955. She still remembered the advice received during her lectures from many years before and planned an efficient, labour-saving day over a very early breakfast.[113] When one is cycling from one end of a large parish, or even several parishes, it is a good idea not to cover the same road more than is absolutely necessary.

For most nurses, the first duty of the day was visiting people with diabetes. They had to have their injection of insulin before breakfast. All of the nurses interviewed remember the early-morning list of injections. This was a seven-day-a-week task and, where possible, neighbouring nurses tried to allow each other a Sunday morning off by occasionally doing another district in addition to their own.

Mary Quain's student notes of 1936 offer an insight into the quantity of work that had to be done in the ordinary day of a Queen's nurse. These notes, in condensed form, recommend visiting difficult midwifery and maternity cases in the morning, after the diabetics. Acutely ill and new patients who would be 'unduly apprehensive' should then be seen. Those surgical cases requiring twice-daily dressing would be next on the list. Chronic cases, blanket baths and supervisory or casual visits should be fitted in as convenient, and infectious cases, including those with tuberculosis, should be left until as late as possible. The evening visits were effectively a repeat of the morning schedule, covering those who required a second visit. Then there would be the extra visits. Very ill patients required a third visit during the day or, for instance, usually, a mother who had recently delivered exhibiting a raised temperature. Penicillin, it seems, in 1936 had to be administered intra-muscularly three times a day. Any late-night visits were exclusively for emergencies or for those who were on morphine injections (the terminally ill), and regulations for its administration were strictly adhered to. It was advised that families of patients should be asked to do some of the nursing duties on Sundays but there would always be the unavoidable injections and acute cases that nurse must attend to even on the day of 'rest'.[114] The rounds were the mainstay of the day around which surgeries, school visits, deliveries of babies, contact with doctors and simply getting from place to place were structured. It shows how little room there was for emergencies such as floods, storms and epidemics. At times such as these, the workload snowballed but still had to be done.

Etta Catterson Smith went on a morning round of South-East Dublin with Nurse Ryan in 1892 to report for the magazine *The Lady of the House.* 'We went speedily from house to house, bandaging, plastering, bed-making and washing, a number of old women principally, until past one o'clock … She was to make a second round in the evening, she told me, upon which she would take up the wants of her male patients who would then be returned from work.'[115] Of these men, she wrote that the nurse treated 'severe scalds among the lead-smelters and glass-blowers, while the fishermen of course endure much cold and get laid up with inflammation of the lungs'.[116]

An easily forgotten part of the rounds was the presence of dogs. Both Maura Kilmartin and her daughter, who was a public health nurse, reminded me of how essential it was to record the name of the family pet so that it may be possible to gain admittance to the home by cajoling the canine security service of your good intentions. Mary Duffy describes bringing her daughter, Delia, to give a regular injection to an elderly lady in the district. The old lady would lock the dog in the bedroom and hold the door fast until Delia would grab the handle and both nurse and patient were then free to medicate. When they were leaving they would prepare and make a quick dash for the door with hound snapping at their heels.[117]

At the end of the day there was the paperwork. The ability of a nurse to keep good records was highly prized by the Queen's Institute inspectors and it was noted several times on nurses' records. Mary Quain, as a trainee district nurse, was lectured on the rationale for recording everything. From the perspective of the individual district nursing association and the Queen's Institute, statistics of the work done were important to justify its demand for support from the public or the local authorities. They also acted as a vital part of the public records of births, deaths and infectious diseases, and for the nurses' own protection against accusations of malpractice. It also helped the nurse taking over a new district if good records had been kept by her predecessor.[118] Mary Quain describes the Jubilee nurse sitting down after her evening meal to fill in the records. These consisted of a general register, a time book, a daily visit book, the Queen's Institute midwifery register, the local authority midwifery register, the TB register, child welfare cards and the donation book.[119] The difficulty was that many of the very active and caring nurses were so busy carrying out their work with their patients that there may not have been much time or energy left at the end of a long day to sit down and record the happenings of the day. It must have taken a great strength of character to develop a habit of daily paperwork. It was certainly not a part of the job which any of the nurses interviewed saw as a pleasure. It was just something that had to be done. Daily notes were scrutinised on the inspection of the district once or twice a year and were available for perusal at all times. We have not yet found an example of one of these case books. They were, in all probability, destroyed deliberately because of the sensitive nature of the material they held.

We do, however, have very tangible specifics about the work done by the Queen's nurses throughout the existence of the scheme. Every nurse in every district counted the number of visits they made and the types of appointments. They logged this information monthly and submitted it, usually in person, to the district nursing association and by post to the Queen's Institute. The records for every district were published in the Queen's Institute annual report and the numbers are quite startling. In 1928 it was possible for Lady Kenmare to record that the average number of visits for each nurse was 4,000 per annum.[120]

With the organisation of a day's round in mind we selected a random year, 1935, and looked at the statistics for a very typical district. Lismore is a rural village in County Waterford and the Jubilee nurse operating in this district in 1935 was Kathleen

Knowles. She made 3,451 nursing visits to ill patients, 1,315 home visits to tuberculosis sufferers and 5,798 public health visits that year. That number records doors opened to the nurse and grateful patients seen, in their homes, for one year. She had 160 surgical and medical cases, many of whom would have called to the clinic for dressings but it is not recorded how many times. That year the nurse only had four cases of midwifery to attend to herself but 4,415 cases for infant welfare and antenatal care. Some of these would have called to the clinic but many were, again, home visits. She made 68 school visits.[121] These numbers varied a little on emphasis of practice in different districts but were characteristic of the work done by individual nurses. Considering there are only 365 days in the year – 30 of which were annual leave – and many districts that year had higher figures including much more maternity cases, it makes one marvel at how they did it. Nurse Knowles stayed in the district until 1945.

DISEASE

The history of diseases, their treatment and vaccinations were intrinsically tied to the changing circumstances of the Queen's nurses. As diseases such as tuberculosis, other epidemics and welfare concerns came into or out of public focus, so the nature of the workload for the nurses in the community changed. Antibiotics had a profound effect for anyone in the business of saving lives. Most of the deadly epidemics were bacterial, and great numbers of healthy young people died of minor injuries due to infections that could not be treated. When penicillin came onto the market it was revolutionary, but Mary Duffy describes giving it intramuscularly domestically, with no backup in case of toxic allergic reaction. She says she was very lucky this never occurred and that it was only given when absolutely necessary.[122]

EPIDEMICS

Queen's nurses normally had very busy practices but in times of epidemic, nursing was calamitous, as can be seen by the description given by Annie P. Smithson in her memoirs of the terrible influenza epidemic that raged all over Ireland in 1918. She succumbed to the disease that was killing people at a drastic rate, took a week off and had to go back before she was fit because there was 'not a nurse to be had for love or money to take my place'.[123]

Nurses were quite helpless in the face of collapsing communities. They rushed from house to house trying to relieve the suffering, and often great loss of life, with nothing in the 'magic bag' but panacea. In the early stages little was known about the causes of epidemics and so there was no effective treatment. Sometimes, as in viral infections like the great flu of 1918, there was and still is no real cure. The nurse simply had to carry on calmly, doing her best to alleviate symptoms, and encourage the family to ride out the fever. It was felt that educating the family members who would attend to patients may contribute to the prevention of death in some cases. Many of the diseases with high fevers required constant care and cooling of the patient by the family, with sudden recoveries and equally sudden deaths. A calm, resourceful Queen's nurse explaining clearly the actions required probably saved many lives over the years. Most of the diseases that caused the epidemics which were dealt with by voluntary district nurses are no longer with us and many do not know, or have forgotten, what they were. For clarity, and because they are a primeval part of our history, the following is a short summary of some of the common diseases named in this chapter.

TUBERCULOSIS

Until the arrival of antibiotics, and for a good decade after, the disease of tuberculosis (TB), also known as consumption, was demoralising. Many of the Queen's nurses had special qualifications as TB nurses or had worked in sanatoria where it was treated specifically. Lady Aberdeen had a special group of Queen's nurses trained as TB nurses, including Annie P. Smithson. It was an enormous part of the workload due to the huge numbers of patients falling ill with it and because the Queen's nurse often ended up treating the whole family, not just the individual. Many of the victims were younger people, often the breadwinner, in a time of very little social welfare. TB did not only afflict those suffering from extreme poverty and hunger but these factors exacerbated the disease and its spread. In 1907 Dr E.J. McWeeney reported to the Statistical and Social Inquiry Society of Ireland (SSISI) that in the battle with TB 'we may well despair of accomplishing anything when we remember that the average labourer in Dublin does not earn enough to maintain a family in a state of physical efficiency'.[124]

Unlike other bacterial infections it did not have a dramatic, epidemic-type nature. It was called the white plague because it was more insipid and slow to kill. It was a confusing disease because for most it affected the lungs with horrible bleeding coughs – this was pulmonary TB. It did also affect all the other organs and particularly, it seems, the bones, which made it difficult to diagnose. In many instances the treatment for this type of disease was the surgical removal of the infected bone. In the early part of the twentieth century TB was beginning to be recognised as a communicable disease. In conditions where whole families lived in one-room tenements there was little a nurse could do to alleviate the risk to all the family members. Florence Nightingale's fresh air and hygiene theories were all very well if one could afford a bar of soap or had heat or access to fresh, clean water. The sterilising formalin lamp suggested by Lady Aberdeen in 1909 may have helped a little. She was also very active in the efforts to distribute pasteurised milk through depots in Dublin.[125]

Streptomycin was introduced as a treatment from 1948, and the BCG vaccination began in 1949. While the numbers affected started to decline after these developments, there were still 3,166 cases of TB in Ireland in 1960 and 468 people died of the disease that year.[126]

Typhus

Typhus was, like TB, a bacterial infection which claimed the lives, or health, of many patients, nurses and doctors alike. It caused a flu-like fever which some recovered from but many did not. Those that recovered could be carriers unknown to themselves. Initially, localised outbreaks would occur and the nurse would fight back by trying to isolate individuals, clean homes and get people to boil their drinking water. The difficulty with the disease, from a nursing point of view, was that it was carried from home to home on the lice that were endemic before proper pesticides. In 1944 a company producing dichlorodiphenyltrichloroethane (DDT) set up in Galway supplying the whole of Ireland. This, along with the schools inspection programme, helped put an end to typhus and its very nasty epidemics.

TYPHOID

Typhoid was also a bacterial epidemic associated with contaminated water and food supplies. The nature of this illness entailed enteric fevers, or a horrible tummy flu from which the individual could die. Again, epidemics would occur in the community. Initially little was known of the reason for these occurrences and even if they did know, the medical people had no laboratory support to help find the source. Nurses continued with their boiling water advice, as well as recommendations that patients should keep homes clean in order to avoid infection of their neighbours. This was advice provided in the case of all epidemics.

DIPHTHERIA

Diphtheria was caused by yet another nasty bacterium. It was a respiratory disease which was spread through the air and sometimes infected people without their knowledge so that they became unknowing carriers. Those it did affect badly, often children, would develop a swollen throat that could prove to be fatal. An emergency tracheotomy was often the only way to save the patient's life. Jubilee nurses were well trained in the skills of emergency tracheotomy because diphtheria was a relatively common disease, and once the wound had healed and the fever abated, many people survived. An immunisation programme was instigated in the early 1930s which effectively eradicated the disease.

POLIOMYELITIS

Polio was a terrifying viral disease which usually affected children. Outbreaks spread fear and suspicion throughout communities. Schools were closed for long periods and many children were kept at home. This was because of the drastic and often fatal nature of the disease. Some badly affected ended up being kept alive in 'iron lungs' because their respiratory systems were temporarily paralysed. Many children were left with permanent paralysis and atrophy of limbs that often required surgery and long years of rehabilitation. This disease still had the power to create pandemonium until the mid-1960s when a proper vaccination programme was instigated in Ireland.

OTHER DISEASES

Smallpox was extinct by the 1920s. Many people will remember outbreaks of, usually non-fatal occurrences of, childhood viruses and scarlet fever, which is the streptococcal bacteria but tends to be a mild illness. Whooping cough, measles, mumps, chickenpox and the usual colds and flu would have affected all communities on a cyclical basis. In the earlier stages of the scheme, when healthy nutrition and adequate clothing were not the norm, these diseases caused great concern for Jubilee nurses. Later they would have been aware of these outbreaks and concerned for some of their more vulnerable patients. All of these diseases are usually mild, but whooping cough, mumps and German measles (rubella) are now part of childhood vaccination programmes. This is because, for several different reasons, they can leave long-lasting side effects on the patients themselves or others they come into contact with.

In 1903 the Marchioness of Waterford in the second annual report for Carrick-on-Suir District Nursing Association congratulated subscribers on having the skilled nursing of Miss Kelly that winter. The gratitude of those who benefited during the severe epidemic of whooping cough, with its attendant complications, was reward enough for their generosity.[127] Anyone who has nursed a small child will know the distress of whooping cough, and as a highly contagious bacterial infection in 1903 it was also fatal for many.

MIDWIFERY AND CHILD WELFARE

Many districts did not require a midwife as there may already have been one employed by the state. However, all Lady Dudley nurses required midwifery training and it was useful to have the skills in every district. Nurses within an area where districts were in close proximity to each other offered help to neighbouring nurses, especially with midwifery cases. This practice was described by Nurse Quain to Therese Meehan.

> Once, when she was waiting with a woman in labour, she had a 'strong feeling' to check in on another woman about a mile away whom she knew had been delivered by a nurse from another district some hours before. At times when several women were in labour at the same time nurses from other districts would try to help one another. Mary found the woman haemorrhaging severely without anyone in the house realising what was happening. She sent urgently for the doctor and priest, massaged the fundus and got the woman into a head-down position. The woman survived and Mary got back to the first woman in time for her delivery.[128]

The Jubilee nurses interviewed from Tramore and Kilmeaden lived locally to their districts, which were in close proximity, and relied on each other to do relief work. While Bridget Hartery had midwifery cases – about one a month – Ann Connolly did not. It was essential she was trained and experienced even though there would have been little opportunity for her to practise the skills. In her first district in Donegal, where she did not practise midwifery, Mary Duffy commented that 'on occasions when the maternity nurse was snowed in I had to deliver babies, once three in one week. Thank God I never lost a mother.'[129]

Maura Kilmartin began domiciliary maternity care in Dundrum when asked to do so by her committee after the previous, council-sponsored midwife died suddenly. Delivery of a baby in the late 1950s cost £1, which was given straight to the district nursing association. Some deliveries could take days. It was an enormous responsibility for Queen's nurses on the district, who had to put all other work on hold while they attended to midwifery cases. Maura Kilmartin remembers having to wait for the doctor after a baby was born with physical defects, before talking to the distressed mother. She brought many babies into the world in her district but she found they were increasingly likely to be problem cases, due to the fact that they had not attended the nearby maternity hospitals for prenatal checks, and it was all becoming too dangerous. She therefore informed her committee that she would discontinue the practice in the early 1960s.[130] Nurse Anna McLoughlin in Manorcunningham supported this view. In later years when she had deliveries they tended to be those of unmarried girls or women who, for whatever reason, had not informed the authorities. As a result, the deliveries were often emergencies and frequently very difficult.

In an interview on 6 September 2011, Dr Áine Sullivan of Cavan said that her father, the dispensary doctor for the area, believed if the doctor was called to a maternity case that was being managed by the Jubilee nurse, it was indeed a great emergency. Professor James Muldowney, a former resident of Bennetsbridge district, now living in Canada, wrote to us to assist our research. He reminisced about Nurse Alice Brady, the Jubilee nurse in attendance in the 1930s, who delivered both himself and another patient on Christmas Day 1939. Both babies were delivered safely despite it being a 'brutal day'. He returned more than 60 years later for a family gathering. A photograph was taken of both 'Christmas babies' with Alice Brady, who was in her nineties, at the time and lived to be over 100. The 'babies' were in their mid-sixties. He said: 'We had to hunt Alice down to take the pictures as she had stepped outside to have a smoke.'[131]

For most Queen's nurses, child welfare formed a very large and important part of their work. However, this was not the case in districts where a state child welfare officer was present – in these circumstances the district nursing association could not apply for the grant to provide this service. There were two grants available to district nursing associations – the tuberculosis grant and the maternity and child welfare grant. The latter covered the cost of maternity and follow-up on deliveries, which included checking the baby and mother and the suitability of the home and ensuring the welfare of all. After an initial period of home visits after the baby was born, the mother was encouraged to visit the welfare centre until the child was five years old for follow-up supervision. These grants in effect covered children through school and also included the inspection of schools.

The development of a state child welfare system in Ireland was slow and patchy. A lecture given to the SSISI in 1911 entitled 'Medical Inspection of Schools and School Children' by

Mr J.B. Story, MD complained that 'medical inspection of school children exists in a more or less complete form in every civilised community except our own'.[132] The main reason why it was (and still is) essential to inspect schools is that it facilitated a subtle way of accessing families and evaluating childhood illness or problems that could be remedied before they became permanent. Eyes and ears, developmental problems and any signs of malnutrition were particularly monitored. It still is the most logical way to administer vaccination programmes. It was a means of preventing the spread of communicable disease including ringworm, impetigo, scabies and other parasites. The other vital part of school inspections was conducted discreetly by the nurse to ensure there were no vermin in the hairs of the children. This was not cosmetic. The transmission of typhus via head and body lice, described above, was rampant in schools. The health visitors to schools in the 1960s, who were not Jubilee nurses, wore a grey uniform and were colloquially referred to as the 'grey ladies' or the 'nit nurses' by locals.[133] In the earlier stages before DDT was banned as a toxic substance for the treatment of parasites, it was administered in the schools or handed out free to the children going home. According to Dr James P. Murray, this policy of dealing effectively with the country-wide louse infestation probably prevented serious outbreaks of typhus in the 1940s.[134]

As part of their training, Queen's nurses received lectures on 'School Nursing'. They learnt the laws governing school inspections and how they evolved. It was the responsibility of the nurse to assist the medical officer in the school visit by ensuring there was appropriate accommodation for the clinic and that record cards were up to date. A Health Visiting Card was created for every baby born in the district. It recorded the first six years of life and it was up to the nurse to ensure it was sent to another district if the child's family moved and to the school when they first attended. She also had to make sure any doctors' recommendations were carried out. To do this she had to visit the homes of children and advise their parents. As part of her responsibilities for the general welfare of the children in the school environment, she conducted regular visits to all the schools and teachers in her district. School medical inspections for each child were supposed to occur at five, nine and at leaving either at thirteen or sixteen years.[135] Miss Quain said she always tried to visit the schools on 'Friday afternoons in order to cause as little disruption as possible. By visiting one school weekly and checking a couple of classes, all the children were checked regularly.'[136]

Mary Duffy in Donegal recalls her memories of the school visits in the district of Newtoncunningham in the 1960s.

> Immunisations were done at intervals in schools. We also had to check children's eyesight, teeth and check for head lice. One mother complained and objected to me checking for head lice, I reported it to the nursing superintendent and then we stopped doing it. Later parents were sent leaflets to inform them if there was an outbreak of head lice. I had to attend six schools, one in Bridgend, Killea, Carrowan, Moness, two in Newtown, one Catholic and one Protestant. Children were much healthier then as they walked to school.[137]

Head lice infection was not the only condition checked for in the schools. In 1909 the *Queen's Nurses' Magazine* had an article titled 'Nursing in National Schools in Ireland' in which a nurse stated that of a population of 300 children, around 24 'would be suffering from the following diseases: Accidents, burns, otorrhoea, eczema, warts, ringworm, impetigo contagiosa, the last two are very contagious, as we all know, and when you see one case you are sure to see more.'[138] An abbreviated version of the nurses' description for the treatment of impetigo was to remove the crusts (soften with a little oil first) and apply a dressing of white precipitate ointment; it alleviates the great itching characteristic of the disease.

Dentists were also sent to the schools to monitor children's teeth before dental problems could develop or to arrest difficulties as they occurred. These visits were also assisted by the district nurse and responsibilities similar to those involved with the medical visits ensued for her.

Lady Aberdeen was dreadfully concerned about the lack of childhood care and high infant mortality in Ireland during her second tenure as the viceroy of Ireland's wife in 1907. She insisted that babies' clubs were set up in all the branches of the Women's National Health Association (WNHA). This valuable service provided a venue where mothers with babies and toddlers could call for advice from the nurse or just to meet others in the same position for mutual support. They offered a cup of tea and a bun to entice the mums to come, and often used the gathering as a chance to hand out clothing and extra food supplements. Catching medical problems early in a baby's life can save them and also prevent unnecessary long-term suffering. A centre where district nurses can weigh and monitor babies, administer early vaccinations and generally advise young mothers is now the norm.

However, this was not always the case, and the district of Dundrum in County Dublin is one example. Child welfare was Maura Kilmartin's special interest. This was particularly useful in a community that had an exploding population when she arrived in 1952. Comparatively, her predecessor, Nurse Jones, had taken an interest in the elderly of the district. By 1946, records for the Baby Club which had been set up by the Women's National Health Association in Dundrum had effectively ceased. In 1952, shortly after her arrival, Maura Kilmartin was 'full of enthusiasm from [her] time in Holles Street Maternity Hospital' and decided to reinstate the baby club concept. Accordingly, she organised a meeting of mothers once a month in the dispensary. The baby club evolved into the present child welfare clinic that is still running in Dundrum.[139]

One of Maura Kilmartin's regular – and enjoyable – work calls was to the Children's Sunshine Home in Foxrock every month. This small residential care unit was built in the 1920s by Dr Ella Webb, with much of the funding received from the Overend Family of Dundrum, to prevent children with rickets becoming permanently disfigured. Rickets was a disease of babies kept in tenement basements who did not get enough sunlight, or vitamin D, for bone development. They were given sunlight treatment, hence the name of the home, and returned to their families after a few months, well fed and with straight legs. Subsequently, discovery of the link with vitamin D eliminated the need to remove babies from their parents for the sun treatment. The home then became a place of accommodation for severely physically and mentally disabled children. As a small unit it has a homely quality but many of the children need comprehensive nursing care on a daily basis. Nurse Kilmartin's job at the time was to ensure the good care was maintained and to offer advice to the staff. Part of this centre is now the LauraLynn hospice, which is a support facility for terminally ill babies and their families.

Not all of Maura Kilmartin's experiences were this positive, however. The care of special needs children was traditionally a deeply neglected, veiled part of Irish society and still was during the 1950s and 1960s. She had not realised the extent of the population of children with special needs in her district until the Government Commission of Inquiry on Mental Handicap began to record statistics from 1961. Parents of these children appeared out of the woodwork when the opportunity arose to secure financial support. Maura Kilmartin began to receive calls from across the district and it upset her that she had never met any of these children before.[140]

The Lady Dudley Scheme had a toy fund in which donations of toys, made and purchased, were distributed at Christmas in districts where there was a nurse. It was in operation from the very early days of the scheme until the late 1960s.[141] It must have been a great joy for the nurses to be part of this distribution of happiness. Photographs from annual reports show children with their small but precious gifts.

THE ELDERLY

In 1925, her committee stated of Nurse Jones in the annual report that 'she was attentive and kind to the sick poor under her care and attended the old and feeble with efficiency and consideration'.[142] This would have been very acceptable to the committee of the Dundrum District Nursing Association because there were many family retainers in Dundrum who had connections to the committee. These family 'retainers' could have been gardeners or groundsmen but were often 'women of gentle birth' who had restricted financial support. Many had worked all their lives as cooks, housekeepers and nannies with the same family and, upon their retirement, often ended up living in dilapidated properties or gate lodges with very little pension. Their care was a concern for these families, but as single independent people it was easier for everyone if the Jubilee nurse looked in on them from time to time. As with child welfare and other care organisations, retirement institutions and homes for the elderly were also part of the visiting duties of the Queen's nurse.

Mary Duffy's district was top heavy with elderly in need of care. Fortunately, her personal focus of interest lay in this area. She describes saying the rosary with two elderly bachelors every evening. In an interview, she and her daughter, who assisted her as a child and went on to become a nurse herself, described extraordinary success in this area. As mentioned above, the nurse could not be with the family all of the time and it was her task to ensure that the urgency of her instructions were understood and carried out. When patients survived catastrophic strokes, or were incapacitated through old age or other debilitating diseases and confined to bed at home, the organisation of their care formed a mammoth task. Essentially, they were under the overall care of the dispensary doctor and his family, all of whom relied on Mary Duffy to support them. In order for a bedridden patient to live for years, and even decades, they had to have a very good diet, plenty of fluids and regular turning to prevent bedsores. Their physical care was a great challenge for the entire team, but to keep a person's spirits up for decades was an even greater feat. Mary mentioned that at one point she had ten stroke victims in her district.[143] That was ten daily visits, ten bed baths, and much discussion of care and the problems that would crop up from time to time, such as chest infections and dehydration leading often to confusion and distress. Support and understanding for the caring family was just as important to the success of the endeavour as the care of the patients themselves.

In 1958 the County Medical Officer in Donegal discussed the very high proportion of elderly living alone in Donegal due to the emigration of the young. He deplored the lack of voluntary district nurses to take care of the elderly, who were otherwise hospitalised. This occurred at greater cost to the state and also meant that individuals died in hospital rather than in their own home, which is what they would have preferred.[144]

The Local Hospital

Sometimes the nurse was no longer able to provide enough care at home and patients were sent to hospital. In the early stages of the

Queen's Institute's presence in Ireland, there was a great fear of being sent to hospital, but even at later times in history it was, for many families, a traumatic event. In many cases, people would delay calling a medical professional until it was very late and their first point of contact at this stage would have been the nurse. Maura Kilmartin described the days before mobile phones and having to run to the nearest phone box to get the doctor or an ambulance. She said that even in her time throughout the 1950s and 1960s, people, particularly the elderly, were terrified of going to Loughlinstown Hospital or Number One James' Street because they were still associated with the poor houses of old. Her attempts to get beds for patients in hospitals were recurrent. She said she had a special relationship with some of the senior staff of the Meath Hospital, where she trained and which was relatively near to Dundrum. Nurse Kilmartin also had a special relationship with St Ultan's Children's Hospital because the local dispensary doctor's wife was a consultant there and they would always find a bed for patients from Dundrum and their mothers. She sensed this was a great advantage in ensuring the best care for the patients she was worried about. Of course, when patients were returned to the district Nurse Kilmartin would continue to care for them at home in a seamless manner.

EQUIPMENT

In the days before plastic wrapping, the biscuit tin was an essential part of the shopping experience for many people and also formed an important part of the Jubilee nurse's inventory of equipment. Some of us will remember that cake, sugar, biscuits, sweets and many other items arrived home from the shops in large lidded square or round tins. In confectionery shops you could get really big square ones. A useful storage container for everyday use for the Queen's nurse, they were a most important piece of equipment. In their kitchens, the nurses would sterilise gauze, lint and 'rolls of gamgee' by baking them in a paper-lined tin in their oven. The lid was left off at first and sealed back on while still very hot to keep the contents uncontaminated for transporting.

The District Nurses' Supply Depot (DNSD) at 14 Merrion Square, Dublin sent bales of surgical dressings all over the country.[145] A

Irish Life, January 28th, 1916.

IRISH WAR HOSPITAL SUPPLY DEPOT.

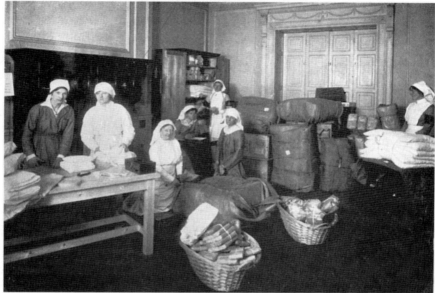

Photograph   THE PACKING ROOM, 40 MERRION SQUARE.   Chancellor, Dublin.
Mrs. Wynne and some of her helpers.

Courtesy of the Airfield Trust, Dundrum.

joint committee of the St John Ambulance and the Red Cross gave an annual grant to fund this distribution. Volunteers offered two days a week to make bandages and dressings. They were thanked annually in the reports of the Queen's Institute. Letitia Overend, representing the DNSD, and her central workrooms committee appealed every year at the annual general meeting for 'gifts of old linen, all kinds, and also for volunteers to help prepare, sew, pack and despatch all the various equipment which was sent to our nurses'.[146]

Patients who required frequent dressings had a biscuit tin in the house to hold their own supply of gauze, bandages, sterilised water, a kidney dish and forceps. Dressings were done for patients who had suffered burns, lacerations and the never-ending varicose ulcers with older patients. The dispensary doctor would recommend the treatment programme to be continued, usually until healing was complete. Many elderly people with varicose ulcers suffered pain and weeping wounds for months and often years with very little sign of healing. Mary Duffy in Donegal recommended some of her elderly patients visit the seaside regularly to walk in the water where the seaweed would brush up against their intractable varicose ulcers. The results were always good and often quite spectacular. Her daughter said in an interview that recent studies of the healing properties of seaweed support the belief in this therapy that Mary Duffy devised herself.[147]

In the days before antibiotics, wounds were very dangerous as sepsis would lead almost inevitably to death. Phyllis Sproule remembered the first effective antibiotics being used in the district. It must have been profoundly gratifying for these nurses to witness the end of so many horrible diseases, such as tuberculosis, and the enormous difference it made as previous treatments were highly ineffective and merely supported the patient's own healing response.[148]

Disposable gloves, needles and syringes were to arrive when there were no more Jubilee nurses. The biscuit tin, once again, was of immense practical value to hold all the tools and requirements for routine injections, particularly those needing insulin. The water and syringe – a glass and chrome affair with large needle – had to be boiled to sterilise it every day. This was done before the nurse left so that it would be cool enough to use quickly in the morning. Methylated spirits were used to clean the skin and kept in a little jar. Nurse Mary Byrne said 'there were a lot of jars' for all sorts of uses, such as holding the needle while you drew up the injection and for sterile water itself. Newspaper was invaluable for keeping working areas clean of everyday dirt in the home and for gathering up used dressings at the end of a procedure. According to an article in the *Irish Nursing News* of 1952 on sterilisation of syringes: 'With regard to the needles, if nurse has not good eyesight she should carry a small watch-maker's lens round with her, so that she may be sure the needle is really sharp.' The needles were, it seems, sharpened on an Arkansas stone.[149]

In 1892 the reporter for *Lady of the House* magazine described the work of Queen Victoria's Jubilee nurses to her readers. 'Each lady carries under her cloak a bag that is better than Fortunatus' purse, for the actual things wanted are found at hand in it, not merely the where-withal to buy them.'[150]

The nurse's bag was a key part of her equipment. An expensive and rather heavy leather item, it went everywhere with her. In April 1932 Miss Colburn of the Queen's Institute wrote to Miss Hart of Carrablagh, County Donegal discussing the setting up of the Fanad Health Club. She asked if they would like her to order official district bags as they could only be sourced in Dublin. By the end of May everything was arranged for two nurses to be sent to this isolated peninsula of north Donegal. They were to take their district bags and necessary books with them. Miss Colburn grumbles that Fannin's, a medical supplies shop, 'sent an account for one nurse's bag only, as two were ordered – but this firm employ the worst book-keeper I ever met, so please do not pay the bills, but send them on to me'. Miss Colburn also suggested buying the bicycles locally as it was easier to get repairs carried out by whoever supplied the bicycle.[151] Many archived photographs of nurses show the bag propped up on the carrier in front of her bicycle. To avoid contamination, it was never allowed to touch the floor. There were several compartments in this bag and the outer one held soap and a towel and newspapers. Equipment was laid out on clean newspaper or on the bag itself, and even the nurse's coat did not come in contact with potentially infected surroundings.[152]

Mary Duffy described the bag in her memoirs. 'The nurse's bag was equipped with dressings, iodine, forceps and bowls which would be boiled in the house where the patient was. Syringe and needles were also necessary. Often they became blunt from reuse and boiling. Iron injections were often given as many of the women were anaemic due to poor nutrition and frequent pregnancies. M and B tablets were given for fevers.'[153] Most nurses had two bags – one for midwifery and one for general use. The contents would have been very different but, more importantly, it was essential not to transfer contagious diseases into the house of a pregnant woman or her newborn baby. Earlier Lady Dudley nurses describe the shock of not having water, or a utensil to hold the water, for the washing of newborn babies.

Annie P. Smithson said of her time in her first district in 1901: 'Every night I had my surgery when patients would come for dressings or advice, many of them sent to me from the doctor, who was glad to have this help.'[154] Of course the bag had to be restocked,

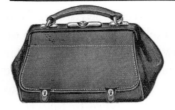
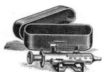
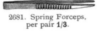
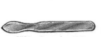

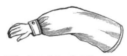
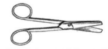

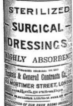
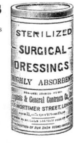
Courtesy of Queen's Nursing Institute, London.

often twice a day, and the store for this was normally kept in the nurses' clinic. Most nurses had their own small clinic, usually in their front room. They would have done dressings for ambulatory patients and given immunisation injections or carried out doctors' requirements dispensing medicines, often, in the early stages, compounding them also. In some cases the nurse's clinic was in fact the dispensary doctor's clinic as well.

We take for granted a lot of convenience today with regard to routine medical supplies. In 1906 the annual general meeting of Cork District Nursing Association was recounted in the *Queen's Nurses' Magazine*. Nurse Baxter read her report: 'She mentioned what a boon the gift of knitted bandages was to a district nurse.'[155] One could presume she was hoping to encourage the practice of hand-knitting bandages among the people of Cork. Today, individuals go to the pharmacy and, without prescription, can attain a specific ointment in a tube for all sorts of skin lesions, itches, rashes, wounds and bruises. Jubilee nurses made up an ointment that was a catch-all cure for every skin problem. Mary Quain's recipe for 'Queen's Ointment' was taped to the front page of her student notes in 1937. It was made from one and a half pounds of lard, three quarters of a pound of Vaseline, four ounces of zinc-oxide, four drams of carbolic acid and three drams of creosote.[156] Presumably some of this unction was decanted into a small container for carrying around in the bag to be used whenever it was required. The latter two ingredients must have given this a very distinctive aroma – a perfume that was likely to go before, and linger after, the nurse had done her ministrations in every home.

GETTING AROUND

Unlike in the case of hospital work, domiciliary nurses had to call to their patients, many of whom lived in rural areas at the end of long boreens with incessant gates to open and close. Those with inner-city practices had endless stairways to go up and down. The actual task at the end of the journey may only have taken fifteen minutes, but getting there may have taken 40 minutes, or much more, and for some of the island nurses a few hours and imminent risk of death in a currach. Lady Dudley's nurses in the early part of the 1900s sent letters describing the hardship they encountered among their patients; these were published in the annual reports and reveal the great courage the nurses showed. A nurse in Galway in 1908 described how she 'had been to a confinement case to one of the islands since one o'clock this morning. It was so stormy and it took such a long time to get there, I really thought I would never reach it safely. The waves were almost dashing over my head, and of course plenty of salt water to drink. They hadn't got a boat, but a currach, in which I daren't move. I hope I will never experience such a dreadful night again.'[157] Dr Thomas Hickey thanked Lady Dudley's Scheme for sending Nurse Donald to his dispensary district in Spiddal, County Galway in 1903. 'As an example of her zeal, I cannot do better than mention that some time ago she was obliged to go on a certain case and for the journey she rode seven miles (English) on her bicycle and then was obliged to ride on horseback for five miles and finally had to cross a lake in a boat, before reaching the pathway, some 100 yards in length, which led to the house of the patient.'[158]

When interviewing nurses about the dangers of attack in travelling lonely roads, often at night, it was universally agreed that they perceived no danger except that of tripping or falling over on rocky roads. This said, Annie P. Smithson described in her memoirs finding herself on a well-known country road without a bicycle lamp, on a moonless night, cycling in circles. Eventually she heard footsteps and decided to risk asking for help, 'even if it was someone who might murder me for the sake of my clothes and leave me on the roadside stripped naked'.[159] She said she never went out without her bicycle lamp again. Her colourful descriptions did include a few portrayals of the paranormal or ghosts that she encountered on lonely roads, normally towards dusk.

The nurses interviewed gave several accounts of comings and goings and many noted that the local doctor would often be leaving a delivery or clinic at the same time and offer them a ride home. These occasions would be useful in the exchange of concerns or triumphs with regard to mutual patients. Sometimes when a patient's family was sent to get the nurse they would escort, and possibly even drive, the nurse to where the patient was.

In the earlier years of the Queen's Institute in Ireland, the district nursing associations may have provided a pony or jennet and trap for the nurse. Peter Griffin of Kilmeaden, County Waterford remembers his father teaching Nurse Mary Dooley to drive a small Ford van in the early 1950s. He said that before the arrival of the car, transport for the nurse was a pony and trap provided by the president of the district nursing association, Mrs Susan Dawney. He remembers the name of the pony as 'Velikiye Luki', seemingly named after a Russian city that was featured in the Second World War.[160]

In 1963 the minutes of the Lady Dudley's Scheme monthly meeting suggested it was a good idea to give the nurse in Carna driving lessons and that they would cover the expense.[161] For the vast majority of Jubilee and Lady Dudley nurses, however, their main mode of transport was the bicycle. Occasionally they were permitted to hire a hackney carriage or car on days of extreme weather. This extravagance would have been very occasional as most district nursing associations did not have the surplus finances. People who remembered the Jubilee nurse in their district always refer to the big black bicycle as part of that memory. The cost of the bicycle, and its upkeep, was a great expense for the district nursing associations. For the nurses it was imperative that they learn how to ride a bicycle but not everyone did. It was noted on the Roll of Jubilee Nurses whether a nurse was already a cyclist. In 1907 Nurse Henrietta O'Brien qualified as a Queen's nurse and worked in several urban districts until she was appointed to Bangor, County Down. She resigned within a year because she was unable to cycle.[162] Nurse Smithson described her experience as a relief nurse in the North of Ireland being taught to ride a bicycle by the young maid who was employed to cook and clean for her.[163]

Transport by bicycle was not ideal in Ireland, particularly in the west where days of continuous rain and wind made the routine of getting around even more hostile. Mary Quain describes her period of time in Carraroe, County Galway when she would cycle up to 30 miles a day, heading out on visits with the wind against her. The same wind would turn to meet her on her way back. She felt she was always heading into the wind. She told Therese Meehan that the winters were hardest. 'She had five heavy coats but it was not always easy to keep at least one of them dry. Sometimes she had to don a saturated coat and bike miles in cold, lashing weather to attend a woman in labour.'[164]

According to the St Patrick's Nurses' Home annual report of 1949: 'A small motor car was bought in February 1948 and is used by the Staff Nurse in the course of her duties as nurse instructor. As these duties may take her anywhere from Drimnagh to Sandymount, the car has proved a special boon in saving time during the period when so few candidates were available.'[165] St Patrick's Home was still, at that time, located at 101 St Stephen's Green. The reference above was to the difficulties encountered in getting enough candidates trained to fill the vacancies in the country.

Mary Byrne said her father lent her the money in the late 1960s to buy a Ford Anglia to travel her district in Naas.[166] In many cases the acquisition of a car would have seemed a very desirable improvement in conditions, but in some districts this may not have been so. Mary Quain explained that she got a car in 1939 but gave it up because she found that, instead of easing her work, she ended up doing more walking. This was because at the beginning of each homestead there would be a gate to keep in livestock, followed by a pot-holed, rocky mud track to the house.[167] Mary Duffy acquired a car in 1949, when her brother went to a show at the Royal Dublin Society (RDS) in Dublin and bought a Ford Anglia for £400. Before the purchase of her car the district nursing association committee of Manorcunningham, County Donegal under the leadership of Mrs Chance organised a rota of farmers and their wives to drive the nurse about on her afternoon visits after the clinic.[168] Many nurses remember the scooter that was eventually provided by the committee. In November 1963 the Lady Dudley's committee discussed Nurse Foley in Glencolmcille and the fact that she had a scooter but was given permission to hire a car for travelling in bad weather.[169] Maura Kilmartin, who paid £14 for her own bicycle on the day she left the Meath Hospital, was grateful to Mr Joe Daly, the man who serviced her bike. He fitted a little motor to help her up the many steep hills of Dundrum village. She went through three of these motorbikes before the district nursing association closed down.[170]

LIVING CONDITIONS OF THE NURSE

'Down by the water's edge, in lonely state, stood a whitewashed cottage with a slate roof. A high whitewashed garden wall, reached to the eaves, seemed to grow out of the side walls of the cottage, and protected a pretty little garden alike from relentless winds and inquisitive sheep.'[171] This was the description of Nurse O'Dowd's house in Fanad district in 1935 on an isolated peninsula in north Donegal.

Most nurses had a good house, relative to the general population, and frequently also benefited from home help. This was a prerequisite of setting up a district nursing association and remained an important factor for continued affiliation. The superintendent's inspections were directed at both the nurse and the committee itself in this regard. An emphasis on the provision and maintenance of suitable accommodation was fundamental in the organisation of district nursing from its inception. Florence Nightingale, co-founder of the Queen's Institute and highly influential in the early development of the nursing profession, said of the home of the district nurse that if the nurse is 'to set these sick people going again, with a sound and clean house, as well as with a sound body and mind' the organisation must provide 'a home fit for her to live in'. With regard to help in the home, 'if a nurse has to "find herself" to cook for herself when she comes home "dog tired" from her patients, to do everything for herself, she cannot do real nursing.'[172] The nurse's accommodation was seen as an opportunity to lead the people by example. As the Countess of Mayo said in 1924: 'Such houses not only shelter our nurses, but also serve as an object-lesson to the people, many of whom have no idea of how a decent house ought to be kept.'[173] The didactic nature of the Jubilee nurse's work and the importance of her living a clean and healthy life in a suitable home cannot be overemphasised. The Jubilee nurse belonged to the community and reflected its aspirations.

Many district nursing associations began by offering salary inclusive of board, lodging and laundry, or two rooms, fire, light and attendance. Standards, such as the provision of two suitable rooms, were strictly adhered to. Often a house was rented in a central location within the district. Several associations began with an affluent member of the committee, usually the president, purchasing or building a cottage for the nurse. This small house or cottage was then furnished by members of the committee. Even when the nurse had her own front door she still had to ask her committee for permission to have relatives to stay for a holiday. Other 'guests' were not even considered. When an established district provided a cottage, often by a new committee, it was included in the list of affiliated branches of the Queen's Institute and was seen as a gesture of strong intent to continue the work. The provision of a cottage or private house for the nurse became more important with the introduction of telephones as boarding houses were less keen to provide a messaging service along with the nurse's laundry and meals.[174]

Annie P. Smithson began as the first nurse in her first district in Gilford, County Down in 1901 and stayed for three and a half years. Her home was on the main street beside the police barracks of the small village. Annie noted in her memoirs that her house was comfortably furnished. She had the usual surgery room on the ground floor off the main hall, as were the kitchen pantry and coal shed which was stocked with a ton of coal and a supply of wood. Upstairs were her own sitting room and bedroom and the next floor contained two bedrooms – one for the maid and a spare room for guests. A full-time maid had been hired for her from the mill where almost everyone else in the village was employed. The work was, like many country districts, demanding but Annie's memories of that period often included 'sitting by the fire in my sitting-room'.[175]

Mary Duffy (nee Kearns) began in the district called Taughboyne, otherwise known as Carrigans, County Donegal in 1948. She describes her arrival in her unpublished memoir:

At that time nurses were appointed by local committees and I was asked to come and work in Donegal to cover for the local nurse who had pneumonia. I left Dublin by train for Donegal in 1948. I was met by Miss J.K. Baird at Carrigans Station and I was taken to the nurse's cottage in Carrigans and settled in there. The cottage was donated to the Nursing Association by the McClinock Family, Dunmore. The cottage was on the Main Street, it had two rooms – kitchen and like all homes then, it had no running water or light. Dry toilet outside. Open coal fire. There were two telephones in the village, one in the

Post Office and one in the Garda Barracks. At that time there were few cars.

Miss Baird was the secretary of the district nursing association that was set up in 1941. Initially the association had offered the first nurse lodgings, assuring the Queen's Institute that this situation was temporary. By today's standards the house, the cottage donated by the McClinnock family would not exactly be seen as the lap of luxury, but for postwar, edge of Europe it was not bad. Tucked in beside a small church and rectory, the house has now fallen into disrepair (planning permission for its demolition is being sought) but is still a wonderful example of vernacular housing in a small village.

In interviews, Maura Kilmartin described her accommodation in Dundrum as very unsuitable in the beginning. Her predecessor, Nurse Jones, had been in occupation for 35 years and bought her own house in the area. The committee did not, as a result, have accommodation for the new nurse. Maura Kilmartin, just qualified, was put into cold, damp lodgings where she remembers being hungry most of the time. Mrs Mulvey, a member of the committee, on becoming aware of the conditions organised the furnishing of a more comfortable apartment over the Bank of Ireland in the middle of the village. Later, Mrs Mulvey, who was an elected county councillor, arranged for one of the new council houses in Mulvey Park, Ballinteer be allocated to the Jubilee nurses. The second nurse, Mary Killalea, lived in Mulvey Park because by this time Maura Kilmartin, nee McLoughlin, had acquired a home near the village with her husband.

The Lady Dudley's Scheme usually provided a cottage for the nurse and this, in several cases, was built and maintained by the Congested Districts Board.[176] Mary Quain described arriving in Achill Island in 1943 and being helped by the old woman who had originally helped the first nurse to unpack in 1904. She still did not have running water or electricity.[177] By 1953 their maintenance was becoming a priority, as recounted in that year's annual report. 'The year has not been without its difficulties and anxieties trying to maintain the standard of comfort to which we feel our nurses are entitled. Every effort is made to supply their wants and to keep their houses in as good condition as possible.'[178] The minutes of the meetings of Lady Dudley's Scheme from around this time show how undeveloped a territory the west of Ireland still was. The secretary of the scheme reported in the minutes in 1962 that the previously mentioned 'Nurse Foley of Caherdaniel had visited the office while on holidays, and asked if she might have a bathroom installed. Lady Olein Wyndham Quinn mentioned a local contractor who would do the job at a reasonable price and said she would try to contact him.'[179] In 1963 Nurse Foley got electricity installed. The Lady Dudley's nurse on Inisheer Island was instructed to arrange proper sanitation and running water to her cottage in 1971. The nurse's house in Swinford, County Mayo needed a new cement floor in 1968 in order to keep the rats out.[180] These cottages were still the responsibility of Lady Dudley's Scheme in 1974 when it was closing down. Most of them had become quite run down and in need of repair and were a burden to the committee. In many of the Jubilee districts they evolved into the 'health centre' or were used to offset losses at the closing down of the district. A number are still the responsibility of the Queen's Institute.

Several district nurses were accommodated in the local cottage hospital and had dual responsibilities for nursing patients both in the hospital and the local district. Many of these were in the North of Ireland and examples can be seen in the districts of Cushendall and Bushmills, County Antrim and Coleraine, County Derry. The nurses of St Patrick's Home, Dublin were 'distressed at not being able to get their child patients into the country, began collecting in order to start a little home for convalescent children on the outskirts of the city'.[181] With the generosity of Lady Albreda Bourke they set up Cheeverstown House in Clondalkin, County Dublin. It was to provide fresh air and sunlight to prevent children from inner-city squalor developing permanent physical deformities from rickets. For those whose parents had died of TB it was an orphanage. Two Jubilee nurses lived in the home and were in charge of the ten children normally resident. It operated in this manner from 1905 to 1927 and ten Jubilee nurses were recorded in the list of affiliated associations.[182] Valentia Island in County Kerry and Ramelton, County Donegal also had a village hospital where the district nurse resided.

Later Jubilee nurses remembered their homes with affection. Nurse Fennelly, the last nurse in the district of Cashel, County Tipperary remembers living in a 'chimney shaped' three-storey house, which was only one room wide, in the middle of the town over the dispensary. It had a brass plaque saying 'Nurse's House'. The provision of a cottage or house in the village preordained that the nurse had a small surgery in the front room. At Rush/Lusk in County Dublin, the two nurses who served the district from its opening in 1954 to its closing in 1962 lived over the dispensary. Dressings and injections of ambulant patients could be carried out and advice sought in neutral terrain. In some cases this was also the surgery for the dispensary doctor. The nurse could take routine clinics if required and work at home when they were not so busy. The difficulty with this arrangement was that people saw the nurse's home as an extension of her work practice and not a place she could retreat for rest. As Mary Duffy remarked in interviews, the nurse's home was the centre of care for the people in Manorcunningham and they would therefore call morning and evening. Delia, Mary's daughter, said that the people had begun to queue for her at the door of their home as she was going out in the mornings to drop the children to school. Dr Pippett in Wicklow also noted that irrespective of what they did, the people would not let Mary Kiernan retire. People still called to her home at all hours of the day and night long after she had ceased employment as a Jubilee nurse.

Nurse Connolly in Kilmeaden said she was considered by the committee to be too young to occupy the very pretty nurse's home in the village and stayed in 'digs' for her period in the district. The nurse's house was sold when the district nursing association ceased and is now an antique shop.[183] As living conditions for the rest of the population improved, the didactic nature of the nurse's accommodation became less important. Many of the Lady Dudley's cottages, and several other houses, lived in on a long-term basis by nurses, were purchased by the nurses themselves at the end of the scheme or on their retirement. The last nurse in Birr, County Offaly was able to acquire the nurse's cottage under the 'house purchase scheme' from the Urban District Council.[184]

Most of the earlier Jubilee nurses had help in the home, described as 'attendance' in many of the entries of the list of affiliated branches. In 1907 Grange Con, County Wicklow provided a furnished cottage and the nurse's salary included servants wages, board, etc.[185] Glendermott in Derry provided a furnished cottage for the nurse in 1920 in addition to a ton of coal, wood, oil and charwoman. It could be assumed that, as president of the committee, Lady Florence Beresford was probably responsible for most of those expenses.[186] It was a great burden for district nursing associations to provide a comfortable home environment for the nurse. She was required to remain single and worked such unsocial hours that, for most nurses, assistance in the home was a basic necessity. Jenny Ledingham remembers visiting her aunt, who was the Jubilee nurse for Enniskillen, County Fermanagh in the 1930s, and recalls the presence of full-time help in the house.[187] In 1904 the *Queen's Nurses' Magazine* gave a three-page account from a Queen's nurse in a district in the west of Ireland – she signed herself 'Fuzzy Wuzzy'. The piece, a harrowing account of the conditions of the people, ends with an emphasis on the importance of home comforts for the nurse herself. 'With a cheery "God speed ye, Alannah, and bring ye safe home" ringing in my ears, I mount my bicycle and start my lonely ride of perhaps seven, eight or even nine Irish miles, through bog and mountain, arriving at my comfortable lodgings in due time, where I am happy to see a bright fire burning and either my dinner or a nice hot cup of tea awaiting me.'[188]

At the start of the scheme, the provision of a maid was relatively inexpensive. As the twentieth century modernised, central heating, washing machines and electric kettles took the place of a full-time maid and committees were not in a position to raise extra funding for a nurse's home help.

In the 1930s Mary Quain was provided with a two-bedroom house which had a surgery in the front hall. A coal range was used for heating and cooking and light was provided by paraffin oil lamps. Mary Quain did not have home help even though her two predecessors had a maid. She sent out her laundry but often became exhausted from the physical nature of her work. In 1936 the Queen's Institute wrote to Miss Hart explaining that it was the 'nurse's own responsibility whether she keeps a maid or a charwoman'. Miss Hart had just managed to get the local council to build her nurse a new cottage and wondered what the normal arrangement was with regard to this expense.[189]

The main reason the Queen's Institute preferred unmarried women as district nurses was that they were available to work 24 hours a day. A great deal of support was required for a nurse with children. Rita Pearson, a nurse in the Donegal district, had to pay for home help following her husband's death as she had four children to care for in addition to her work. Maura Kilmartin's mother came to live with her when she returned to work after marriage. Being a Queen's nurse was a demanding career, and juggling the needs of the sick in an entire community with those of your own family took extraordinary organisational skill and commitment.

The Queen's Institute inspector worried for the nurse in the Lady Dudley district of Dooks, County Kerry who came to them in 1952 and had to leave reluctantly for marriage in 1953. She came back, described as an ex-Jubilee nurse, three nurses later with her own home. In 1963 the inspector noted she was expecting a baby but the work was not acute so she was managing. In June 1966, the inspector was concerned for the nurse, who now had six children and no housekeeper, as the district was a very busy one. The inspector returned again in December 1966 when there was an outbreak of measles and the nurse still had no home help. The district closed that month.[190]

Nurses were not allowed to accept donations of money, however in many districts, gifts of fruit, vegetables, fish or the odd can of milk were dropped off at the nurse's cottage from time to time. Jenny Ledingham of the Crumlin district remarked that it was impossible to refuse a packet of biscuits 'to thank the nurse'.[191] Matthew Ganly, a neighbour of Nurse Agnes O'Grady in Ballinasloe, County Galway, remembers his mother asking him to bring water from the local pump to the nurse's cottage. Mary Duffy from Donegal also remembers bringing water back from the well and gathering rainwater in a barrel beside the house. The district committee for Dundrum, County Dublin had traditionally provided fresh milk and vegetables to the nurses in previous decades. However, it was no longer a practice in Dundrum by the time Maura Kilmartin arrived in the district in 1952. The committee occasionally invited

Maura Kilmartin to dinner but had no real understanding of her difficulties. Her salary did not cover an adequate diet, and she often went without meals, despite an extraordinary physical workload and daily cycling all over the district. Occasionally shopkeepers in the village would insist that she take some food when they saw how strenuous her work was and how pale her complexion.[192] In 1952 there were still shortages after the war in Europe and food was scarce and expensive for everyone.

In Naas, County Kildare in the late 1960s around Christmas time Christmas pudding, mince pies and port wine was offered to the nurse on all her visits.[193] This may sound lovely but it was imperative that patients and their families, who had taken such trouble, were not insulted and it was impossible to eat everyone's offering. Mary Duffy of Newtowncunningham, County Donegal refused even the ubiquitous cup of tea for fear of being seen to favour one family over another. She also believed that acceptance of the offering may be seen as a lax approach to her work. She describes the difficulties of preparing food for herself in Carrigens, County Donegal in 1948. 'On my arrival a new gas oven was bought. Many a weekend I would bake soda bread with rations, only to be called

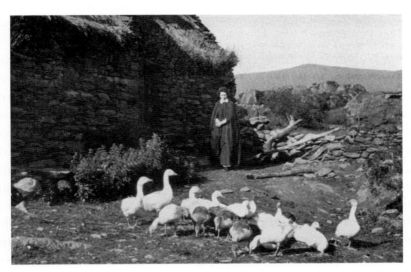

NURSE WALSHE AT GLENGARIFF.

Courtesy of the National Library of Ireland.

out to see a patient, even when I was off duty. I was always on call, my bread would be burned when I returned.[194]

Many nurses grew their own food, as can be seen in Annie P. Smithson's description of her situation in County Mayo in the severe winter of 1916–1917. 'I shall never forget digging a path to the hen-house to rescue my poor fowl.'[195] She kept hens and goats and had her own pretty garden. This was not unusual as it offered an example of good home management. The West of Ireland Association describes in 1905 how 'an original but welcome present was given to the nurse, namely, two ridges of potatoes, oats and grass for the nurse's pony were also given by friends'.[196]

The presence of a companion pet, particularly a dog, was an important feature of the living conditions for some Jubilee nurses. Matthew Ganly of Ballinasloe describes Nurse O'Grady as always having her little dog running beside the bicycle. Upon its death, he buried one of her canine companions in ground surrounding a monument near her home.[197] Annie P. Smithson described making a pet of a seagull with a broken wing in her district in County Mayo. Her black cocker spaniel became rather famous due to the occasional mention in her writings of 'Judy'. Fans of Annie Smithson's books even wrote letters to the dog.[198] Mary Kiernan's dog was named Sandy and he went everywhere with her as she carried out her duties in Wicklow town. While the trainee nurses lived in 'digs', Miss Morgan, one of the last superintendents for the Queen's Institute, lived in St Patrick's Home, Morehampton Road, Donnybrook, Dublin with her dog.[199] The reality was that many Jubilee nurses never married and the company and security of a pet was accommodated by the Queen's Institute.

RELINQUISHMENT

The attitude of the Queen's Institute to nurses who married was unambiguous in the early days of the scheme as, at this stage, they simply had to leave. While there must have been a certain element of joy for the nurse who was leaving for marriage, it would have been tinged with the problem of securing her replacement, particularly if she had been a popular nurse. The marriage of Nurse Christina Sweeney to Lord Stewart in County Donegal was proclaimed, in both the nurse's records and at the beginning of the Roll of Jubilee Nurses, as 'Now Lady Stewart'.[200]

In periods when there were fewer trained nurses than required, the departure of nurses due to marriage proved an insurmountable problem and many married women would quietly slip under the radar and continue to work as 'temporary' nurses. In the district nursing association ledger their name would appear as 'temp' retirement, in some cases many years later. In 1963 the Lady Dudley Committee was asked by the local priest to employ a Queen's nurse who had recently married the manager of a local factory. It did appoint her, but only temporarily, because 'it is not our policy to employ married women and when an unmarried nurse was available a new appointment would be made'.[201] Married nurses were not recorded on the Roll of Queen's Nurses. Drumholm, County Donegal received Nurse Dora Black from Arklow, County Wicklow in 1918. She retired in 1920, on marriage, but returned as Mrs McVitty in 1927 and continued as the Jubilee nurse until 1954. That was 36 years of involvement and care in the same community. There was, however, a large question over pension entitlements for most of these women. In 1966 there were great concern noted in the annual report of the Irish Nurses Organisation. 'Enquiries have been made from the Queen's Institute as to the basis on which they had recommended pensions for Jubilee Nurses, having special regard to the absence of marriage gratuity and the fact the married nurses give such long service in a temporary capacity.'[202]

Not all nurses felt it fair that they were asked to leave on marriage and the patients were often also very disgruntled. Whether a nurse was allowed to stay after her marriage depended on the attitude of the individual district nursing association committee and how hard it was prepared to campaign for its nurse to continue. Peter Griffin of Waterford describes the great tension when Mary Dooley married in 1955 and refused to leave the district of Kilmeaden, County Waterford. She had trained as a general nurse and midwife in England and then as a Queen's nurse in St Laurence's Home. Kilmeaden was her first district in 1942, where she received excellent reports from the visiting inspector over the years. They were particularly impressed with her record keeping. After her marriage there was a boycott in the area and people refused to attend the nurse that was appointed as her replacement. Peter Griffin says that despite her great friendship with Nurse Dooley, his mother, who was on the committee, supported the Queen's Institute rules on the subject. The institute accomplished its objective in this case, with the new nurse remaining.[203]

Maura Kilmartin met her husband Mr Kilmartin, the vice-principal of the national school in Dundrum, County Dublin when she carried out a school inspection in her first year as a Jubilee nurse in that district. There was, she said, a regulation that you were not permitted to marry for two years after qualification. On marriage she went to the superintendent in Leeson Street to offer her resignation, when she was told: 'Good news – the regulations have been waived for you.' She continued as a married Jubilee nurse for four years until she became pregnant with her daughter in 1961. She took leave of absence when her daughter was born, until the Queen's Institute wrote to her asking her to return to her post when her daughter was four years old. Her mother came to live with her and she was able to continue until she retired. Maura Kilmartin had a very close working relationship with the Queen's Institute because Dundrum was near to the city and it was easy to drop in. She attended annual meetings with her committee and would have met with all the management staff of the Queen's Institute. She said that she had a significant personality clash with Miss Quain over the years and they disagreed over various matters. She felt that in reality Miss Quain could not reconcile herself with the idea of a married Jubilee nurse.

One of the qualities that made a good Queen's nurse was flexibility, and this led to several nurses leaving their districts for work abroad. Many left for Canada and Australia, where they were qualified to work as Queen's nurses. The US, England and wherever the Irish diaspora was to be found was a destination for several. The support of a religious community appealed to many Queen's nurses and was a socially acceptable option in conservative Catholic Ireland during the twentieth century. Their departure, for this reason, was recorded by the Queen's Institute as 'nurse left for convent'.

During times of war in Europe many nurses answered the call to service and requested leave from their districts, some temporarily, to assist in the war effort. The Great War of 1914–1918 claimed numerous nurses, with some districts losing several to the same conflict. The Second World War attracted fewer district nurses. The qualifications and independent minds of Queen's nurses made them valuable assets in times of stress and social disorder. The numbers of nurses who left districts in Ireland in the mid-1940s were increased by those who joined the United Nations Relief and Rehabilitation Administration.[204] Founded before the United Nations, it was established in 1943 to administer the diverse measures that were supporting victims of war in many countries. Providing shelter, food and medical needs for 'displaced persons camps' in Europe and Asia, it had the support of 44 nations and cared for eight million refugees. The Queen's Institute replaced all of these nurses and welcomed them back after their tours of duty.

Many nurses died while still employed on the district, such as Nurse Josephine Purcell who died in 1937 after 40 years of giving care with the Father Healy District Nursing Association in Bray, County Wicklow. Agnes O'Grady died after an operation in 1955, leaving her friends on the committee bereft. They were given a temporary replacement but the association closed that year.[205]

Nurses who served over six years were entitled to leaving badges whereas those serving less than six years were only entitled to leaving certificates. After 21 years they received long service badges, bestowed in a special ceremony with a mention in the annual report. When a nurse was leaving she handed in her badge to the Queen's Institute. It was re-issued if she wished to resume her duties. Mary Kiernan did this three times before settling down in County Wicklow.

Nurses leaving to retire, on the other hand, were a cause for great celebration tinged with a little worry over the funding of her pension. The Queen's Institute supported the district nursing association committees by replacing nurses who left, but it was often disappointing to see a committee disband after the loss of a nurse. Approximately 50 nurses practised for between 20 and 30 years. Appendix 1 records some of the more longstanding nurses in districts all over Ireland. Lists of names cannot do justice to the debt of gratitude felt for these nurses by those who remember them.

The Queen's Institute appreciated the cordial working relationships developed in communities where the nurse remained at her post for decades. The benefits were tinged with the realisation that some nurses became set in their ways and refused to modernise. As a professional institute that was aware of the improvements in medicine, it still had not created a mechanism for in-service courses. There were a few exceptions, with scholarships – particularly for midwifery – or TB training. In Northern Ireland in 1947, grants were given to several nurses including one to Miss Ledingham for a refresher midwifery course.[206] It was assumed that the annual one or two-day visits of the Queen's Institute inspector would suffice to advance knowledge. The problem was that they also had to supervise the committee, the quality of nurses' housing, the records the nurse kept and in addition had to go on rounds with her. This time was too occupied for anything but rudimentary discussion of improvements that could be made. Towards the end of the scheme the inspectors themselves were becoming rather set in their ways. Voluntary district nurses had very little genuine free time or spare finances. It would have taken a very dedicated nurse indeed, to have the energy after a day's cycling and hard physical work, to acquire books and study in the evenings.

Later nurses noted that there was, in fact, little professional support for Jubilee nurses compared with that available to the public health nurses. Nurse Connolly and Nurse Hartery worked in two adjoining districts in Kilmeaden and Tramore, County Waterford and helped each other out to organise off-duty time and occasional maternity cases. Without this support they would have been on call all the time, with no break except for annual leave. The isolation and responsibility was bound to take a toll on the emotional and physical welfare of nurses. The Queen's Institute was aware of this problem and felt the solution was that, once a district was established, the committee would be responsible for the physical and emotional support of the nurse. In many instances this was the reality. Of course, this was not always the case and as such, transfers were arranged and a more suitable fit was made between committee and nurse. Towards the end of the scheme, Jubilee nurses were state-registered professionals and not as dependent on what they often perceived as the unqualified busy-body interferences of their committee.

HEALTH

District nursing was a hazardous occupation until the later part of the twentieth century with the introduction of effective anti-biotics. A nurse's health was considered her own responsibility and an extremely important one in her line of work. The training of nurses emphasised hygiene and preventative measures the nurse should take, but it was accepted that many nurses would contract some of the diseases that were endemic in the population. The *Queen's Nurses' Magazine* reported regularly on the welfare of nurses. In December 1905 it noted that 'Nurse Farrelly and Nurse Donald both have contracted typhus while in discharge of their duty, but we are glad to be able to report that Nurse Farrelly is now quite well again, and Nurse Donald is convalescing.'[207] Lady Dudley, in the same magazine, discusses Nurse Donald's absence from work due to contracting typhus as a very personal regret to herself, 'but it serves today as a reminder of the devotion to duty and the spirit of self-sacrifice which has characterised all along the work of the nurses under the scheme'.[208] Nurse Josephine Bird suffered from typhus fever in 1904 after five years serving Oughterard District Nursing Association, County Galway. She was sent to Castlebellingham, County Monaghan, Valentia, County Kerry and eventually her health broke down in Celbridge, County Kildare. Celbridge was very sorry to lose her in 1925 but she was no longer able to care for such a large district.[209]

Nurse Armstrong in Dooks, County Kerry recovered from typhoid in 1914 but the very popular Nurse Neeson in Fairymount, County Roscommon was not so fortunate. The Lady Dudley Scheme discussed the women in its annual report. 'These two cases show how necessary it is to insist on the nurses maintaining a certain standard of living. Therefore how impossible it is to reduce expenditure in that direction.'[210]

In many instances a single nurse dealing with epidemics in the community with little support was deeply distressed by the plight of her patients and working around the clock. Accordingly, it was inevitable that she would become run-down and succumb to the infection, thus being unable to help her patients when most needed. As described by Nurse Smithson, who was working in Milltown,

Dundrum and Clonskeagh district through the famous flu epidemic of 1918: 'The influenza was frightful. I was on duty night and day. I saw four in a bed often – all very ill. Next day one would probably have died. On the last day that I was on duty before collapsing myself, I had visited 35 cases.'[211] Annie had five years previously been sent to the recently opened Peamount Sanatorium for the treatment of tuberculosis in her right lung. She had contracted the disease during her time as one of Lady Aberdeen's special tuberculosis nurses in the TB dispensary in Charles Street, Dublin.[212]

Mary Byrne in an interview discussed the dangers of contagious diseases and said the nurses simply could not afford to think about them. They took all precautions possible but had to carry on visiting despite outbreaks of infectious ailments. She remembered vividly an outbreak in Crumlin, Dublin of infective hepatitis where whole families came down with jaundice. She also mentioned that scabies, head lice and worms were another worry for a nurse visiting people in their homes.[213] Of course many of these parasites had their own mobility and while there was a treatment at the time it was often very harsh on the patient and nurse if she contracted them.

Both Nurses Mary Byrne and Phyllis Sproule remember the problem of fleas or, as they called them, 'hoppers' when visiting the residents of inner-city Dublin during their training and work in St Patrick's Nurses' Home. These itchy bloodsuckers, while a constant problem, seemed to outbreak in waves, normally during the summer, and avoiding them was almost impossible. The nurses lived in 'digs' and would have to treat themselves with DDT, a potent and now banned chemical, when they returned home in the evenings.[214] A vile concoction with 'pripsen' (also no longer available) was the treatment for worms, and children were regularly dosed on the assumption that they had them.

In many instances, even the most resilient women found rural districts too strenuous. A heavy midwifery practice had to be juggled with school inspections, visits and dressings for the sick and old, along with dealing with epidemics in all weathers. This workload took its toll on a nurse's physical health. Often the annual inspection would be a chance for the Queen's Institute to assess how well a nurse was managing, and if there were indications of health trouble she would be transferred to a less busy district. This was the case for Mary Quain, who was transferred from Carraroe in west Galway which was, at the time, the heaviest midwifery district in the country. She described in a lecture in 1987 the strain of her workload. 'There were 75 to 80 home deliveries each year. It kept me on the move all the time; there was no possibility of working regular hours. Indeed on some occasions, a week passed without even getting to bed. At the end of the week it was not surprising that one was exhausted.'[215] Miss Bourke, the Queen's Institute inspector, decided to offer her a less busy practice in another Lady Dudley's district at Keel Village, Achill Island, County Mayo.[216]

In 1910, an article in *Sláinte* for the Women's National Health Association discussed the problems of stress faced by district nurses. The reality was that some communities had a nurse and others did not, hence disease eradicated in one area was waiting in the next parish to return. They were also dealing with grave poverty and, with no proper social welfare, families starved if the father did not go to work, even if he was dying of TB. 'The utter helplessness of district nurses to render any but temporary aid in half the cases which they attend is at the root of the nerve exhaustion and depression which often attacks the most devoted workers.'[217]

The Affiliated Nursing Associations lists record death as the reason for leaving a district in at least eight instances, but not what the death was. It is therefore not possible to state how frequently nurses were the victims of accidental death. Kathleen O'Connor was nurse for Waterville District Nursing Association in County Kerry from 1920 to 1928 and her 'reason for leaving' was because of accidental death.[218] Many accidents were caused by the fact that some nurses had enormous territories to cover by bicycle. While roads were less busy in the early part of the twentieth century, they were also potholed and irregular for cycling. There were many incidents recorded, such as the following from the *Queen's Nurses' Magazine* in May 1906.

> Miss Dowling, Queen's Nurse at Castleknock, met with a serious bicycling accident on May 14th. A party of bicyclists collided with her at cross-roads, with the result that she fell and fractured her leg. Dr Pim happened to be passing and had her conveyed to Rathdown Hospital. Miss Dowling is, however, now convalescent.

Not everyone recovered from these bicycle accidents and many had to leave the Queen's Institute altogether following an accident. Even when an accident was not fatal it could take a long time for a woman to recover her confidence. The Queen's Institute inspectors noted with alarm how dishevelled the nurse in St Anne's district, Iniscarra, County Cork had become in 1949 after an auto-cycling accident. Before her accident she was 'well liked and hard working' but afterwards was 'rather untidy and inclined to grumble'. She left later that year to get married but returned as the 'very capable' last Queen's nurse in Cork city.[219] As road traffic increased and nurses used cars more frequently there was also the inevitable risk of car accidents. Moycullen, County Galway had a district nursing association from 1919. In 1963 its nurse was left with permanent injuries as a result of wounds she sustained in a car accident while on duty. However, she continued to work in the district until it closed in 1967.[220]

Along with infectious diseases and the possibility of accidents, isolation was another great strain which led to unhappiness and much difficulty for the Jubilee nurse and, more particularly, the Lady Dudley nurses. Their isolation was noted in 1906 when Lord and Lady Aberdeen visited some westerly districts because 'these nurses, who live in such remote and barren districts, inhabited only by their patients and the parish priest, must indeed welcome visitors such as these and must appreciate this evidence that, buried away as they are, they and their work are not forgotten by those in the outside world'.[221]

Annie P. Smithson asked for a transfer from Glencolmcille in County Donegal, her third district. She describes coming from Dublin and city life to the great isolation of the north-west. She felt she had little in common with the people, whom she did not understand. Having struggled on for eighteen months, she gave up suddenly. 'I stared out at the broad Atlantic, at the great cliffs shelving down to it, and at the mountains all around. I thought of the angry storms – such storms as I had never known before – which I had been through in the two winters I had spent there, and I felt that I could not go through another like them.'[222]

CRUSADERS

As advocates for social change and improvement, Queen's nurses were often the outsider in the community that could focus the people on actions that would improve, in a practical way, the lives of many. One of the first examples is not one of our featured Jubilee nurses, but worth mentioning. Born to an English aristocratic family in 1861, the Honourable Albinia Broderick trained as a district nurse in England. She found herself in Cove, Caherdaniel, County Kerry in 1905 and tried unsuccessfully to found a hospital and, with more success, an agricultural cooperative. The dreadful poverty she witnessed – 'the children haunted by tuberculosis, the women tortured in childbirth, the men struck low before their time'[223] – drove her to dedicate all of her property and the rest of her life to the care of the people in this small district in south Kerry. The Lady Dudley's Scheme, with the help of the community, supported nurses in Caherdaniel from 1906 until 1966.

Many Queen's nurses went way beyond their normal, rather full, day's work to relieve people who they perceived were in need. Meals on wheels was an example of this. It is now a vital voluntary service in most towns and many villages which offers the elderly or incapacitated a full dinner once a day. Rita Pearson of County Donegal recalls persuading her district nursing association committee to call a public meeting to form a new committee to set up the service. She had heard about the idea and realised that, in a rural area with a very high elderly population, it would be life-saving. She was in Dublin on private business and went to Drumcondra, where the service was founded, to find out how it could be set up elsewhere. The committee was initially not convinced of the need but under persuasion from Mrs Pearson decided to give it a go. The association celebrated its fortieth year of meals on wheels a few years ago.[224]

Mary Kiernan of Wicklow, who had a particular interest in the elderly in her area, had begun to cook meals and distribute them long before the concept of meals on wheels had begun. She also purchased a nebuliser herself to use when called to emergencies of respiratory conditions where this would be of immediate relief before admission to hospital. While in the district of Kilcoole,

County Wicklow she set up the Kilcoole Music Festival in 1955. It is now one of the oldest events of its type and runs for six days, with 50 competitions of a staggering variety and age range of competitors. Wicklow is a seaside town and Mary Kiernan was aware of the many retired single seamen in her area. In the days before mobile phones, she distributed foghorns and the distress horns of seafarers so that the elderly could call her, or their neighbours, in times of emergency.[225]

During her time with the Dundrum District Nursing Association, Maura Kilmartin was instrumental in assisting a group of people to establish a telephone support service for parents throughout Dublin, initially referred to as 'Parents Under Stress'. This service line is still in existence today as Parentline, which operates under a model similar to that of the Samaritans and offers support to parents who are struggling to cope with their responsibilities.[226]

Finola Smyth, the newly qualified Lady Dudley's nurse in Arranmore Island, County Donegal in 1968 organised a fundraising project to provide a launderette for the island. She contacted the parish priest and had the cooperation of fifteen ladies on the island to run the service. It was provided free to the elderly and incapacitated and all others were charged. The main difficulty for Nurse Smyth was raising the money to erect the laundry and the £146 required for the washing machine. She began a door-to-door collection and a raffle and called to the head office of Lady Dudley's Scheme in Dublin to ask if old sheets and a sewing machine could be sent to the island as part of the project. Miss Quain told her there may be a possibility of a grant from the county council for the building.[227] This young woman, distressed by the unnecessary hand-washing of clothes and sheets by the women in her district, could not allow it to continue. It was characteristic of many of these nurses that she cajoled and organised people and ultimately got things done.

On a simple human level these nurses were also chosen as godmothers to countless children. It was a way of formally honouring them as great role models and a significant way of rewarding their commitment. The examples of specific stories in this chapter are, undoubtedly, the tip of the iceberg. In every community that had a Jubilee nurse there will have been stories of a heroic woman who went beyond the normal duties to assist and care for those in need. These additional services, which were of great benefit to the people, were pioneered by the Jubilee nurses and often became institutionalised, gradually raising the standard of care received by patients.

SOURCES

Sources for this chapter are principally based on the Roll of Jubilee Nurses and the list of Jubilee Affiliated Branches. Both sets of manuscripts, in several volumes, are in the care of An Bord Altranais in the archives of University College Dublin.[228] Another source is the *Queen's Nurses' Magazine* which was published by the Queen's Institute. Contributions from nurses in Irish districts, and articles concerning them, were published in this magazine until the Irish branch of the Queen's Institute was set up. These magazines are catalogued and available in the Queen's Institute Archives in London. The annual reports of the Queen's Institute in Ireland included details of the placements and transfers of Queen's nurses but rarely had space for narratives of their work or lives. Letters from district nursing associations to various organisations such as the local county councils and health officers occasionally illuminated conditions the nurses worked in. All are now in the National Archives. Memoirs of relevant Jubilee and Lady Dudley nurses which proved to be very informative include those of Annie P. Smithson (1873–1948) and Nurse B.M. Hedderman (published in 1917), both of which describe life for Jubilee and Lady Dudley nurses in the early decades of the twentieth century. An interview that Therese Meehan, retired lecturer in the history of nursing at University College Dublin, conducted with Nurse Mary Quain as an older woman recalling her experience as a Lady Dudley nurse describes life and nursing in 1930s Carraroe, County Galway. Mary Quain also wrote an article for the *Irish Nursing News* in 1955 titled 'A Day in the Life of a Jubilee Nurse'. Nurse Quain's student notes from her period in St Laurence's Home have been valuable additions to an understanding of the life and experience of Queen's nurses.

Finally, many interviews were conducted with former Jubilee nurses and with individuals who knew Jubilee nurses personally. These interviews, conducted by both authors, represent an invaluable contribution to our understanding of the very significant impact these women played in communities all over Ireland. Many of these women continued to work in the public health system, which was evolving, and brought their discipline and the ethos of the Queen's Institute into the later Irish community care structure.

Former Queen's nurses who were interviewed include Phyllis Nelson (nee Sproule) and Mary Byrne (nee Catherine Mary McGuinness) on 29 April 2010. They spoke of their experiences in Tullamore. Jenny Ledingham was interviewed on 2 September 2010 while she was on holidays in Ireland from Anglesey, Wales. On 12 November 2010, three former nurses from the south-east were interviewed together. They are Bernie Hartery (nee Coleman), Phyllis Fennelly (nee Meally) and Anne Connolly (nee Barry). On 8 June 2011 the authors visited Dr Vincent Pippett of Wicklow. He spoke in depth about Mary Rita Kiernan who had been the last Jubilee nurse in Wicklow town. Michael and Kate Chance organised a group interview to discuss the Newtowncunningham District Nursing Association, County Donegal on 11 August 2011. Among the participants of this meeting were former Jubilee nurse Anna McLoughlin and her daughter Catherine. We were invited to visit Mary Duffy (nee Kearns) in her home in nearby Newtowncunningham, County Donegal. We talked at length with her, and her daughter Delia, and looked at relevant personal documents on 27 September 2011. Mrs Duffy had, with her granddaughter, already created a short document of her memoirs. We have an extraordinarily detailed and interesting account of life and work for a Jubilee nurse from Mrs Maura Kilmartin (nee McLoughlin) in both telephone interviews and a meeting in her daughter's home in October 2011. Mrs Kilmartin was one of the last Jubilee nurses in Dundrum, County Dublin. Following our visit to Donegal, Mrs Rita Pearson contacted us with an extensive telephone interview on 27 October 2011. She trained as a Jubilee nurse in England and worked in Antrim before being offered the last post as Jubilee nurse in Taughboyne, County Donegal.

NOTES

1   Miss Michie, 'Address to the General Nursing Council, 13 February 1920', *The Journal of the Statistical and Social Inquiry Society*, p. 50. National Library, Dublin.

2   Sir Edward Coey Bigger, MD, 'Public Health and Medical Services', in William G. Fitzgerald (ed.), *The Voice of Ireland* (Dublin: John Heywood Ltd, 1924), p. 356.

3   Interviews with Maura Kilmartin, July, August and October 2011.

4   St Patrick's Home, Annual Report, 1896, p. 7. National Archives, Dublin.

5   Margaret Damant, 'A Biographical Profile of Queen's Nurses in Britain 1910–1968', *The Social History of Medicine*, vol. 23 (Oxford: Oxford University Press), pp. 586–601.

6   B.N. Hedderman, *Glimpses of My Life in Arran* (Bristol: John Wright & Sons, 1917). Nurse Hedderman noted, in her memoirs, that the people of the middle island, Innisman, were a distinct people, and spoke a different dialect of Gaelic from the other two islands. The first of the Aran Islands to receive a qualified Queen's nurse was Inisheer in 1934 and Innisman and Innismore received their Lady Dudley nurse in 1936. Jubilee Nurses, Affiliated Branches, P220/30. An Bord Altranais Archives, University College Dublin [hereafter UCD].

7   Therese Meehan, 'Heading into the Wind: A Jubilee-Dudley Nurse Midwife in West Galway from 1937 to 1943', in Gerard M. Fealy (ed.), *Care to Remember: Nursing and Midwifery in Ireland* (Cork: Mercier Press, 2005).

8   Pamphlet published for Queen Victoria's Institute for Nurses, 1913. The Queen's Nursing Institute Archives, Wellcome Library, London.

9   Jubilee Nurses, Affiliated Branches, P220/28–30, vols 1, 2, 3. An Bord Altranais Archives, UCD.

10 *Handbook for Queen's Nurses, by some Queen's Inspectors*, 1924, p. 30. The Queen's Nursing Institute, London.

11 Annie P. Smithson, *Myself and Others* (Dublin: The Talbot Press, 1945), p. 160.

12 Vera Matheson, 'Report of the Discussion after the Lecture "The Nurse and the State" by N.M. Falkiner, MD', *The Journal of the Statistical and Social Inquiry of Ireland* (1920), p. 57. National Library, Dublin.

13 Meehan, 'Heading into the Wind'.

14 QVJIN, Annual Report, 1929, p. 9. National Archives, Dublin.

15 *Queen's Nurses' Magazine* (May 1908), The Queen's Nursing Institute, London.

16 Miss F.H. Aylward, 'Domiciliary Nursing and Public Health Work', *Irish Nursing News* (December/January 1955), p. 4.

17 *Queen's Nurses' Magazine* (1905), pp. 101–2. Queen's Nursing Institute, London.

18 Ibid.

19   Ibid.

20   Annie P. Smithson, *Her Irish Heritage* (Dublin: The Talbot Press, 1918), p. 46.

21   Ibid., p. 54.

22   Ibid., p. 47.

23   Interview with Bernie Hartery, Phyllis Fennelly and Anne Connolly in Waterford, 12 November 2010.

24   Interview with Phyllis Nelson and Mary Byrne, Tullamore, Co. Offaly, 29 April 2010.

25   Maura Kilmartin, interviews July, August and October 2011.

26   *Queen's Nurses' Magazine* (1905), pp. 101–2. The Queen's Nursing Institute, London.

27   Interview with Bernie Hartery, Phyllis Fennelly and Anne Connolly in Waterford, 12 November 2010.

28   St Patrick's Home, 13th Annual Report, 1889, p. 9. National Archives, Dublin.

29   Ruth Barrington, *Health Medicine and Politics in Ireland 1900–1970* (Dublin: Institute of Public Administration, 1987), p. 134.

30   *Evening Mail*, 21 August 1953, Department of Health files, M100/150. National Archives, Dublin.

31   Mary Quain, unpublished notes of lectures on the course for the Queen's Institute, 1937. Pages not numbered.

32   Ibid.

33   Sheila Pim, 'Jubilee Nurses Past and Present', *Irish Times*, 2 March 1966, p. 8. Irish Times Archives.

34   Interview with Phyllis Nelson and Mary Byrne, Tullamore, Co. Offaly, 29 April 2010.

35   Interview with Bernie Hartery, Phyllis Fennelly and Anne Connolly in Waterford, 12 November 2010.

36   Roll of Jubilee Nurses, vol. 4, P220/30–4. An Bord Altranais Archives, UCD.

37   Interview with Bernie Hartery, Phyllis Fennelly and Anne Connolly in Waterford, 12 November 2010.

38   *Handbook for Queen's Nurses, by some Queen's Inspectors*, 1924, p. 30. The Queen's Nursing Institute, London.

39   Smithson, *Myself and Others*.

40   Annie P. Smithson, *Carmen Cavanagh* (Dublin: The Talbot Press, 1921), p. 11.

41   *Queen's Nurses' Magazine* (1916), p. 55. The Queen's Nursing Institute, London.

42   QVJIN, Annual Report, 1947, p. 8. National Archives, Dublin.

43   Lady Dudley's Scheme, Annual Report, 1921. National Library, Dublin.

44   Lady Dudley's Scheme, Annual Report, 1924, p. 7. National Library, Dublin.

45 Miss Mary Quain, address given at the centenary of the Queen's Institute in Belfast, 27 November 1987.

46 Annie P. Smithson, *The Marriage of Nurse Harding* (Dublin and Cork: Mercier Press, 1989, p. 25.

47 Interview with Bernie Hartery, Phyllis Fennelly and Anne Connolly in Waterford, 12 November 2010.

48 Hedderman, *Glimpses of My Life in Arran*, p. 83.

49 *Queen's Nurses' Magazine* (1904), p. 67. The Queen's Nursing Institute, London.

50 Ibid., p. 66.

51 Florence Nightingale, *On Trained Nursing for the Sick Poor*, 1881 (pamphlet). The Queen's Nursing Institute, London.

52 William L. Micks, *The Congested Districts Board for Ireland, 1891–1923*, (Dublin: Eason & Son Ltd, 1925), p. 10. The Congested Districts Board was set up in 1891 by Mr Arthur Balfour, who was chief secretary for Ireland, to provide suitable industries to the poorest counties of Ireland. All of them were along the western seaboard. It was closed in 1923 with the setting up of the Irish government and its functions divided up to their respective ministries. The board had a flexible programme and was essentially there to improve the lives of the people in these destitute areas. William Micks was involved from the very beginning and assisted the new government in its dissolution. He was one of two paid employees in the history of the board and was intrinsically involved in most of its projects. Ibid., p. 91.

53 Ibid., p. 91.

54 Smithson, *Carmen Cavanagh*, p. 129.

55 Smithson, *Myself and Others*.

56 Miss FitzGearld Kenny, 'The Nursing of the Poor', letter to *The Irish Homestead Magazine* (18 February 1901), p. 126. Subscribers to *The Irish Homestead Magazine* sponsored two nurses in the west of Ireland.

57 Miss Michie, 'Address to the General Nursing Council, 13 February 1920'.

58 Meehan, 'Heading into the Wind'.

59 Ibid.

60 Interview with Phyllis Nelson and Mary Byrne, Tullamore, Co. Offaly, 29 April 2010.

61 Lady Dudley's Scheme, Annual Report, 1907, p. 18. National Library, Dublin.

62 Roll of Jubilee Nurses, vols 1–7, P220/37. An Bord Altranais Archives, UCD.

63 Ibid., and Jubilee Nurses, Affiliated Branches, P220/28–30. An Bord Altranais Archives, UCD.

64 Sheila Pim 'A District Nurse's Day: Work, Work, Work', *Irish Times*, 6 November 1955, p. 8. Irish Times Archives.

65 Bangor District Nursing Association, Annual Report, 1905, p. 5. National Library, Dublin.

66   Smithson, *Myself and Others*, p. 162.
67   Ibid., p. 240.
68   Roll of Jubilee Nurses, vol. 1, P220/31, p. 29. An Bord Altranais Archives, UCD.
69   Smithson, *Carmen Cavanagh*.
70   Roll of Jubilee Nurses, vol. 2, P220/32, p. 238. An Bord Altranais Archives, UCD.
71   Jubilee Nurses, Affiliated Branches, P220/29, vol. 2, p. 331. An Bord Altranais Archives, UCD.
72   Smithson, *The Marriage of Nurse Harding*, p. 27.
73   Group interview in the home of Mr and Mrs Chance, Manorcunningham, Co. Donegal, 11 August 2011.
74   Interview with Bernie Hartery, Phyllis Fennelly and Anne Connolly in Waterford, 12 November 2010.
75   Minutes of Lady Dudley's committee monthly meetings, September 1971, M104–100. National Archives, Dublin.
76   Form T.5. Queen's Institute of District Nursing in Ireland. Personal property of Mrs Mary Byrne.
77   Roll of Jubilee Nurses, vol. 6, P220/36, p. 156. An Bord Altranais Archives, UCD.
78   Pim, 'Jubilee Nurses Past and Present'.
79   Interview with Phyllis Nelson and Mary Byrne, Tullamore, Co. Offaly, 29 April 2010.
80   Smithson, *Myself and Others*.
81   Lady Dudley's Scheme, Annual Report, 1911, p. 10. National Library, Dublin.
82   Lady Dudley's Scheme, Annual Report, 1911, p. 10. National Library, Dublin.
83   Smithson, *Myself and Others*, p. 226.
84   Interview with Phyllis Nelson and Mary Byrne, Tullamore, Co. Offaly, 29 April 2010.
85   Interviews with Maura Kilmartin, July, August, October 2011.
86   Interview with Mary Duffy and daughter Delia, Newtowncunningham, Co. Donegal, 27 September 2011.
87   Queen's Institute of District Nursing Form A.2/11.31. Suggested constitution and rules for a district nursing association in affiliation with the Queen's Institute. Found in Miss Hart Box P27/10, Donegal Archives, Lifford, Co. Donegal.
88   Mary Quain, unpublished notes of lectures on the course for the Queen's Institute, 1937.
89   Meehan, 'Heading into the Wind'.
90   Jubilee Nurses, Affiliated Branches, P220/29, vol. 2, pp. 175–375. An Bord Altranais Archives, UCD.

91   Jubilee Nurses, Affiliated Branches, P220/28, vol. 1, p. 241. An Bord Altranais Archives, UCD.

92   Lady Dudley's Scheme, Annual Report, 1916. National Library, Dublin.

93   Miss Michie, 'Address to the General Nursing Council, 13 February 1920'.

94   QVJIN, Annual Report, 1947, p. 19. National Archives, Dublin.

95   Ruth Barrington, *Health Medicine and Politics in Ireland 1900–1970.* (Dublin: Institute of Public Administration, 1987).

96   James P. Murray, *Galway: A Medico-Social History* (Galway: Kenny's Bookshop, 1994).

97   *British Medical Journal* (27 January 1906), p. 227.

98   Carrick-On-Suir District Nursing Association, Annual Report, 1903. National Library, Dublin,

99   Group interview in the home of Mr and Mrs Chance, Manorcunningham, Co. Donegal, 11 August 2011.

100   Interview with Mary Duffy and daughter Delia, Newtowncunningham, Co. Donegal, 27 September 2011.

101   Smithson, *Myself and Others*, p. 185.

102   Ibid., p. 188.

103   Ibid., p. 191.

104   Smithson, *Carmen Cavanagh.*

105   *The Kildare Observer*, 29 November 1902, p. 7.

106   Mrs William O'Brien, *My Irish Friends* (London: Burns, Oates & Washbourne, 1937).

107   Minutes of Lady Dudley's Monthly Meetings, May 1968, M104–100. National Archives, Dublin.

108   Smithson, *Carmen Cavanagh*, p. 151.

109   Dr Vincent Pippett interview, Wicklow, 7 June 2011.

110   Interview with Bernie Hartery, Phyllis Fennelly and Anne Connolly in Waterford, 12 November 2010.

111   Aylward, 'Domiciliary Nursing and Public Health Work'.

112   Quain, unpublished notes of lectures on the course for the Queen's Institute, 1937.

113   Mary Quain, 'A Day in the life of a Jubilee Nurse', *Irish Nursing News*, (December/January 1955).

114   Quain, unpublished notes of lectures on the course for the Queen's Institute, 1937.

115   Etta Catterson Smith, 'A Day in the Life of a Jubilee Nurse', *The Lady of the House* (14 April 1892), p. 24.

116   Ibid., p. 23.

117   Interview with Mary Duffy and daughter Delia, Newtowncunningham, Co. Donegal, 27 September 2011.

118   Quain, unpublished notes of lectures on the course for the Queen's Institute, 1937.

119 Address given by Miss Mary Quain at the centenary of the Queen's Institute in Belfast, 27 November 1987, p. 6.

120 Lady Kenmare's Foreword to the QVJIN Annual Report, 1928. National Archives, Dublin.

121 QVJIN, Annual Report, 1935. National Archives, Dublin.

122 Mary Duffy, unpublished memoirs, Newtowncunningham, Co. Donegal.

123 Smithson, *Myself and Others*, p. 239.

124 Dr E.J. McWeeney, 'Popular Endeavour against Tuberculosis: Its Instruments, Methods and Results', *The Journal of the Statistical Social Inquiry Society of Ireland* (1907), p. 91. National Library, Dublin.

125 Women's National Health Association Annual Report 1909, PRIV1212WNHA/6/1. National Archives, Dublin.

126 Brendan Hensey, *The Health Services of Ireland*, (Dublin: Institute of Public Administration, 1972), p. 109.

127 Carrick-On-Suir District Nursing Association, Annual Report, 1903. National Library, Dublin.

128 Meehan, 'Heading into the Wind'.

129 Mary Duffy, unpublished memoirs, Newtowncunningham, Co. Donegal.

130 Maura Kilmartin interviews, July, September and October 2011.

131 Professor James Muldowney, email letter from Canada, 31 May 2011.

132 J.B. Story, Esq MB, *The Journal for the Statistical and Social Inquiry Society of Ireland*, p. 523. National Library, Dublin.

133 Interview with Jenny Ledingham, 2 September 2010.

134 Murray, *Galway: A Medico-Social History*.

135 Quain, unpublished notes of lectures on the course for the Queen's Institute, 1937.

136 Address given by Miss Mary Quain, at the centenary of the Queen's Institute in Belfast, 27 November 1987, p. 6.

137 Mary Duffy, unpublished memoirs, Newtowncunningham, Co. Donegal.

138 *Queen's Nurses' Magazine* (1909), p. 106. The Queen's Nursing Institute, London.

139 Interviews with Maura Kilmartin, July, September and October 2011.

140 Ibid.

141 Lady Dudley's Scheme, Annual Reports, 1911 and 1968. National Library, Dublin and Donegal Archives, Lifford, Co. Donegal, respectively.

142 Dundrum District Nursing Association, Annual Report, 1925. Airfield Archives, PP/AIR; OPW/NUI Maynooth Archive.

143 Interview with Mary Duffy and daughter Delia, Newtowncunningham, Co. Donegal, 27 September 2011.

144 Annual Report of the County Medical Officer, Donegal, 1958, p. 40. Donegal Archives, Lifford, Co. Donegal.

145 The War Hospital Supply Depot in 14 Merrion Square, Dublin was set up to collect from district depots all over the country, especially boggy parts, bales of sphagnum moss (an absorbent padding for infected wounds)

and bandages, to be made into suitable dressings and despatched all over Europe during the First World War. Miss Letitia Overend was involved in the packing department from the very early stages. Airfield Archives, PP/AIR; OPW/NUI Maynooth Archive.

146   QVJIN, Annual Report, 1935, p. 12. National Archives, Dublin.

147   Telephone interview with Delia Duffy, 14 September 2011.

148   Interview with Phyllis Nelson and Mary Byrne, Tullamore, Co. Offaly, 29 April 2010.

149   Professor Cruickshank, 'Sterilisation of Syringes', *Irish Nursing News* (February–March 1952), p. 10. National Library, Dublin.

150   Catterson Smith, 'A Day in the Life of a Jubilee Nurse'.

151   Correspondence between Miss Hart, Portsalon, Co. Donegal and QVJIN, Dublin, 23 May 1932, Box P27/10. Donegal Archives, Lifford, Co. Donegal.

152   Interview with Phyllis Nelson and Mary Byrne, Tullamore, Co. Offaly, 29 April 2010.

153   Mary Duffy, unpublished memoirs, Newtowncunningham, Co. Donegal.

154   Smithson, *Myself and Others*, p. 174.

155   *Queen's Nurses' Magazine* (1906), p. 19. The Queen's Nursing Institute, London.

156   Quain, unpublished notes of lectures on the course for the Queen's Institute, 1937.

157   Lady Dudley's Scheme, Annual Report, 1908, p. 12. National Library, Dublin.

158   Lady Dudley's Scheme, Annual Report, 1904/5, p. 4. National Library, Dublin.

159   Smithson, *Myself and Others*, p. 183.

160   Peter Griffin, email letter from Dooneen, Co. Waterford, 31 May 2011.

161   Minutes of Lady Dudley's Committee Monthly Meetings, September 1963, M104-100. National Archives, Dublin.

162   Roll of Jubilee Nurses, P220/31, p. 123. An Bord Altranais Archives, UCD.

163   Smithson, *Myself and Others*.

164   Meehan, 'Heading into the Wind'.

165   St Patrick's Nurses' Home, Annual Report, 1949, p. 6. Private collection of the authors.

166   Interview with Phyllis Nelson and Mary Byrne, Tullamore, Co. Offaly, 29 April 2010.

167   Meehan, 'Heading into the Wind'.

168   Group interview in the home of Mr and Mrs Chance, Manorcunningham, Co. Donegal, 11 August 2011.

169   Lady Dudley's Committee, Minutes of Monthly Meetings, M104/100. National Archives, Dublin.

170   Interviews with Maura Kilmartin, July, August, October 2011.

171   'In Wildest Donegal', *The Nursing Mirror and Midwives Journal* (12 October 1935), p. 28.

172   Nightingale, *On Trained Nursing for the Sick Poor*, p. 3.

173   Countess of Mayo, 'Trained Nurses for Rural Districts', in W.G. Fitzgerald (ed.), *The Voice of Ireland* (Dublin: John Heywood Ltd, 1924), p. 363.

174   QVJIN, Annual Report, 1947. National Archives, Dublin.

175   Smithson, *Myself and Others*, p. 186.

176   Countess of Mayo, 'Trained Nurses for the Rural Districts'.

177   Address given by Miss Mary Quain at the Centenary of the Queen's Institute in Belfast, 27 November 1987.

178   Lady Dudley's Nursing Scheme, Annual Report, 1953, p. 6. National Archives, Dublin.

179   Minutes of Lady Dudley's Monthly Meetings, September 1962, M104/100. National Archives, Dublin.

180   Ibid., 1968.

181   *Queen's Nurses' Magazine* (1904), p. 6. The Queen's Nursing Institute, London.

182   Jubilee Nurses, Affiliated Branches, P220/28, vol. 2, pp. 583–4. An Bord Altranais Archives, UCD.

183   Interview with Bernie Hartery, Phyllis Fennelly and Anne Connolly in Waterford, 12 November 2010.

184   Birr Castle Archives, documents setting out terms for Nurse McEvoy.

185   *Queen's Nurses' Magazine* (1904), pp. 19–20. The Queen's Nursing Institute, London.

186   Ibid., p. 9.

187   Interview with Jenny Ledingham, 13 August 2010.

188   *Queen's Nurses' Magazine* (1904), p. 68. The Queen's Nursing Institute, London.

189   Correspondence between Miss Hart, Portsalon, Co. Donegal and QVJIN, Dublin, 29 July 1936, Box P27/10. Donegal Archives, Lifford, Co. Donegal.

190   Jubilee Nurses, Affiliated Branches, P220/29, vol. 1, pp. 475–8. An Bord Altranais Archives, UCD.

191   Interview with Jenny Ledingham, 13 August 2010.

192   Interviews with Maura Kilmartin, July, August and October 2011.

193   Interview with Phyllis Nelson and Mary Byrne, Tullamore, Co. Offaly, 29 April 2010.

194   Mary Duffy, unpublished memoirs, Newtowncunningham, Co. Donegal.

195   Smithson, *Myself and Others*, p. 232.

196   *Queen's Nurses' Magazine* (1905), p. 49. The Queen's Nursing Institute, London.

197   Interview with Matthew Ganly, Ballinasloe, Co. Galway, 6 August 2010.

198   Smithson, *Myself and Others*.

199   Interview with Jenny Ledingham, 13 August 2010.

200   Roll of Jubilee Nurses, vol. 4, P220/34. Directory at the end of the book. Bord Altranais Archives, UCD.

201   Lady Dudley's Committee, Minutes of Monthly Meetings, January 1963, M104/100. National Archives, Dublin.

202   Irish Nurses Organisation, Annual Report, 1966, p. 7.

203   Peter Griffin, email letter from Dooneen, Co. Waterford, 31 May 2011.

204   Jubilee Nurses, Affiliated Branches, P220/28–9. An Bord Altranais Archives, UCD.

205   Interview with Mr Rory Kilduff, Ballinasloe, Co. Galway, 6 August 2010.

206   Queen's Institute, Annual Report from the Northern Ireland Executive Committee, 1947, p. 7. National Archives, Dublin.

207   *Queen's Nurses' Magazine* (1905), p. 92. The Queen's Nursing Institute, London.

208   Ibid., p. 94.

209   Roll of Jubilee Nurses, P220/32, p. 247. An Bord Altranais Archives, UCD.

210   Lady Dudley's Scheme, Annual Report, 1914, p. 9. National Library, Dublin.

211   Smithson, *Myself and Others*, p. 239.

212   This dispensary was initially financed by a New York philanthropist in 1908 in memory of his father, C.P. Collier, and was transferred from management by the WNHA to Dublin Corporation in 1914. Lady Aberdeen, in William G. Fitzgerald (ed.), *The Voice of Ireland* (Dublin: John Heywood Ltd, 1924).

213   Interview with Phyllis Nelson and Mary Byrne, Tullamore, Co. Offaly, 29 April 2010.

214   Ibid.

215   Address given by Miss Mary Quain at the centenary of the Queen's Institute in Belfast, 27 November 1987.

216   Roll of Jubilee Nurses, vol. 4, P220/34, p. 142. An Bord Altranais Archives, UCD.

217   'Nurses and the Public Health', *Sláinte* (May 1910), p. 95. PRIV 1212/WNHA/4/2, National Archives, Dublin.

218   Jubilee Nurses, Affiliated Branches, P220/29, vol. 2, pp. 589–90. An Bord Altranais Archives, UCD.

219   Roll of Jubilee Nurses, P220/36, vol. 6, p. 50. An Bord Altranais Archives, UCD.

220   Jubilee Nurses, Affiliated Branches, vol. 3, pp. 220–30. An Bord Altranais Archives, UCD.

221   *Queen's Nurses' Magazine* (1906), p. 64. The Queen's Nursing Institute, London.

222   Smithson, *Myself and Others*, p. 225.

223   'The Nursing Radicalism of the Honourable Albina Broderick, 1861–1955', *Nursing History Review*, vol. 15 (2007), p. 54.

224 Telephone interview with Mrs Rita Pearson, 27 October 2011.

225 Interview with Dr Vincent Pippett, Wicklow, 7 June 2011.

226 Interviews with Maura Kilmartin, July, September and October 2011.

227 Lady Dudley's Committee, Minutes of Monthly Meetings, May 1968, M104/100. National Archives, Dublin.

228 Roll of Jubilee Nurses, vols 1–4, P220/31–4. An Bord Altranais Archives, UCD; Jubilee Nurses, Affiliated Branches, vols 1–3, P220/29–30. An Bord Altranais Archives, UCD.

CHAPTER 2

The Queen's Institute of District Nursing in Ireland

The Queen's Institute was an organisation which operated across Britain and Ireland throughout the late nineteenth and early twentieth centuries. It was a voluntary body, established in 1889, and was responsible for coordinating the training, supervision and inspection of voluntary district nurses. The Queen's Institute ceased operation in Ireland in 1968 and during its existence it formulated and developed the basis of the modern district nursing service with which we are familiar today.

FOUNDATION OF THE QUEEN'S INSTITUTE

Treatment of disease in the late nineteenth century was a dangerous and difficult task. Hospitals were ridden with infections and often served to exacerbate ailments of the sick, particularly those of lower socio-economic background.

In 1859 William Rathbone, a Liverpool-based businessman and philanthropist, watched as his first wife Lucretia Wainwright Gair received care during her final illness by nurse Mary Robinson. The experience inspired Rathbone to pioneer a system which would offer a similar service to the people of Liverpool who could not afford adequate medical care.

At this time, nursing as a profession was evolving under the strong leadership of Florence Nightingale. In 1860, the first official training school for nurses was opened in London under Nightingale's name. With the assistance and guidance of Nightingale, Rathbone purchased a number of houses across Liverpool throughout the 1880s which served to train nurses, in conjunction with the Royal Infirmary Hospital, in the skills necessary to nurse impoverished

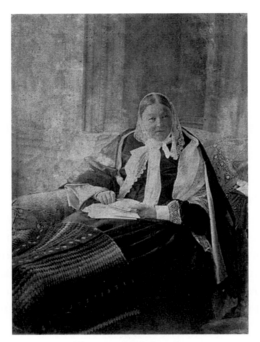

Florence Nightingale.

patients in their own homes. These houses represented the original model of the Queen's Institute's system of training and dispatching voluntary district nurses throughout the communities where their services were desperately required.

In 1887, Queen Victoria celebrated her Golden Jubilee year. In celebration of this occasion, the women of the United Kingdom (England, Scotland, Wales and Ireland) raised a gift to be spent according to Queen Victoria's instruction. This fund amounted to £72,538.17.2 and was entrusted to the Queen to be invested. It was accordingly used to fund the training system recently established by Rathbone and Nightingale 'for the promotion of nursing and the foundation of an Institution for promoting the education and maintenance of nurses for the sick poor in their own homes'.[1] The Queen Victoria Jubilee Institute for Nurses was incorporated by Royal Charter in 1889 and a council was established in 1890. The Queen's Institute was to have its central base in London, with offices in Edinburgh and Dublin. William Rathbone was contracted

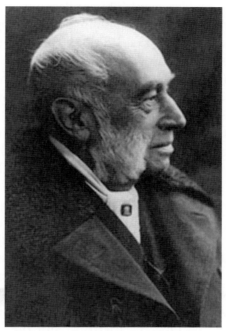

William Rathbone. Courtesy of Queen's Nursing Institute, London.

as the chairman of the sub-committee for organisation of district nursing under the Queen's Institute scheme.

The Royal Charter allowed the trustees to invest the monies raised for the Jubilee Fund at an annuity of 2.5 per cent to be applied in providing improved means of nursing, which extended to the training, support and maintenance of women to act as nurses for the poor and the establishment of homes for such nurses.[2] On satisfactory completion of her training, the name of each probationary nurse was submitted to the Queen as being eligible for entry in the Roll of the Queen's Institute as a Queen's Nurse and would furthermore be recommended for employment as a district nurse.[3]

THE QUEEN'S INSTITUTE IN IRELAND

As William Rathbone pioneered the district nursing service in Liverpool, a group of women in Dublin began to explore a similar concept. In 1876, they established the St Patrick's Home which trained nurses in the provision of care to the people of the poorest parts of Dublin city.[4] This endeavour was supported by the Protestant Archbishop of Dublin (Archbishop William Lord Plunket) and his wife Ann Lee Plunket, also one of the founding members of the St Patrick's Home. St Patrick's Home was first based at York Street but relocated to 101 St Stephen's Green shortly thereafter upon donation of the larger premises by an anonymous benefactor.[5] This house has now been replaced by a modern office block but an article in the *Queen's Nurses' Magazine* in 1905 tells us: 'The Home overlooks St Stephen's Green to the front and has a good view of the mountains from the rear with Lord Iveagh's gardens and the grounds of the Methodist College in close proximity, yet it is situated in the confines of the poorest part of Dublin.'[6]

In July 1888, William Rathbone made contact with Jonathon Hogg, a Dublin merchant who was well connected within the city and was respected by both Catholics and Protestants at the time, with a view to forming a governing body to manage a Dublin-based training school on behalf of the Queen's Institute.[7] Emily Rathbone, William's second wife, took an interest in her husband's involvement with the Queen's Institute and the evolution of the nursing profession and travelled to Dublin to determine whether St Patrick's was a viable option as a training home under the Queen's Institute scheme. It was well established, well managed and served to provide nursing care to the sick poor of Dublin in their own homes. This purpose was much in line with that envisaged by the governing body of the proposed Dublin branch of the Queen's Institute.

According to the thirteenth Annual Report of St Patrick's Home in 1889, its operation was conducted in accordance with the principles of the Church of Ireland, but 'so far as its means will permit, it shall offer its help to the poor of every creed'.[8] This indicated that the home was non-denominational in character, which was correspondent with the ethos of the Queen's Institute that those in need should receive care, regardless of religious belief. Unfortunately, Ireland at that time was encountering political issues related to the British governance of Ireland which resulted in extreme social divisions, particularly on the basis of religious belief. The perception among Catholics in Ireland, following from their experiences of subordination in the eighteenth century, was that people (and women in particular) involved in charitable and voluntary causes tended towards a motive of proselytisation. While St Patrick's Home had the ability to function as a non-denominational training home for the nurses of the Queen's Institute in Dublin, the reigning Catholic archbishop at the time, Archbishop William Walsh, refused to allow Catholic women to live in the same premises as their Protestant colleagues. Equally, the predominantly Protestant governing committee of St Patrick's Home were reluctant to relinquish their autonomy to a Queen's Institute representative committee which would potentially involve the contribution of Catholic members.

A lengthy series of negotiations between the sub-committee of the Queen's Institute (the Dublin Provisional Committee), the trustees of St Patrick's Home and the Catholic hierarchy in Ireland followed Rathbone's initial visit to Dublin. These negotiations were assisted by Lady Ishbel Aberdeen, whose husband had acted as viceroy to Ireland in 1886, and who therefore had a particular interest in Irish affairs.

In search of a solution to the religious conundrum inherent in the use of St Patrick's Home, William Rathbone made contact with two other potential training bodies – the Usher's Quay Nursing Institution, which was governed according to Roman Catholic principles under the supervision of Eliza Brown, and the City of Dublin Nursing Institution which was non-denominational and established by Dr William de Courcy Wheeler in 1883 to train nurses for the hospital in Baggot Street where he worked as a surgeon. Both of these institutions had hitherto nursed only paying patients but both agreed to train nurses for the sick poor on the principles laid down by the Queen's Institute. However, the proposal of an amalgamation of the three institutions under a Dublin-based committee governed by the Queen's Institute was rejected by St Patrick's Home. It became clear to the Dublin Provisional Committee that the ability to implement a system of training of district nurses similar to that pioneered in Liverpool was simply impossible due to the political and religious discord in Ireland at that time. They therefore recommended to the governing body of the Queen's Institute that it should set up an office in Dublin that could supervise the training of nurses, to be carried out within the existing training institutions and homes. This supervising body would have no part in the governance of the homes but would ensure that, upon completion of training, Queen's Institute nurses be dispatched and supervised effectively within relevant communities throughout Ireland.[9]

This arrangement was to change dramatically two years later when, in March 1890, St Patrick's eventually agreed to affiliate with the Queen's Institute. The other two training institutes in Dublin, The City of Dublin and the Usher's Quay Institution, ceased to train probationary nurses when a home was later opened at Mary Street in order to train Catholic nurses. The funds allocated to the aforementioned institutions were then redirected to this home.

First Dublin Office of the Queen's Institute

In June 1889, Mary Lucy Eliza Dunn was appointed to represent the governing body of the Queen's Institute and to supervise the training of nurses in Dublin. Mary Dunn had completed her general nursing and was, at that time, engaged in her maternity training in England. Rosalind Paget, a niece of William Rathbone, was appointed Inspector of Nurses and was responsible for monitoring the work of the nurses upon dispatch to their districts. She later became Dame Rosalind Paget for her contribution to the promotion of women's health and the establishment of the Central Midwives Board.

At this time, Mr and Mrs Rathbone visited Dublin with Mary Dunn in order to introduce her to the principal interested parties and to make enquiries as to where she should reside in Dublin during her tenure. William Rathbone was intent on quickly establishing the working system of the Queen's Institute in Dublin and so Mary Dunn set about finding accommodation in which to live and also to use as an office. She consulted with the Rathbones' existing contacts in Dublin and settled upon suitable lodgings at 14 Nassau Street, located next to a post office and telephone. She commented that 'the outlook [is] nice and tram lines pass the door which would make it easy for the nurses to come to me from their different homes'.[10] The office at 14 Nassau Street was the first address for the Queen's Institute in Dublin.

Through the entire period of this study a very rigorous fiscal control of the office of the Queen's Institute was enforced. Management of nurses, district nursing associations and inspections throughout the whole country was effected with the bare minimum of staff. In later years the office building was shared with Lady Dudley's Scheme. They had separate staff but were able to pool rent and services. Mrs Sheila McCrann, now living in Galway, contacted us with her memories of working in the office at 48 Lower Leeson Street where the Queen's Institute had been situated for many decades. She was employed in the mid-1960s as a shorthand typist to work with Miss Masson who was at the time the secretary for Lady Dudley's Scheme. Beginning straight from secretarial college, aged fifteen, Sheila McCrann said it was a marvellous job that Miss Masson was very kind. She developed a friendship with the other young secretary for the Queen's Institute next door and they would go for lunch together. This office had responsibility for managing the committees' meetings and annual reports as well as the salaries, housing and holidays of numerous nurses in the west of Ireland. They managed it all with a secretary and an assistant of just over fifteen years of age in the days when everything was operated by ledger, letter and post.

DENOMINATIONAL DEFICIT AND THE ESTABLISHMENT OF ST LAURENCE'S HOME

Although training had commenced and the office in Nassau Street had been established as the centre through which the system could operate, Reginald Brabazon, the Earl of Meath, gave an account to the governing body of the Queen's Institute on the progress in Ireland, expressing that there was a problem owing to a lack of properly trained Roman Catholic nurses and until these were supplied the work could make no significant progress in Ireland. This was due to the fact that neither priests nor their people permitted the ministrations in Roman Catholic households of Protestant nurses.[11] An Irish sub-committee was appointed by the Queen's Institute in June 1890. The purpose of this sub-committee was to discuss and attempt to resolve the issue surrounding the requirement of denominational separation. Although William Rathbone had succeeded in bringing the system thus far, the religious complications were making it impossible for the Queen's Institute to progress any further in Ireland.

The primary dilemma regarding the training of Catholic nurses was that accommodation would have to be established separate to that provided by St Patrick's Home. Dowager Lady O'Hagan (1846–1921), widow of Baron Thomas O'Hagan (1812–1885), Lord Chancellor of Ireland, visited Dublin on behalf of the Queen's Institute with a view to formulating a solution to the problem. In her report dated 3 March 1891 Lady O'Hagan states that 'Mr. Charles Kennedy has promised a house rent free, furnished and in good repair with all rates and tax paid, in fact free of charge, for four years subject to the Archbishop's approval'.[12] Mr Charles Kennedy was a close friend of Archbishop Walsh. This house was located at 21 Mary Street, in the centre of Dublin, and described as a 'large old gentleman's house of the last century'. On 1 July 1891 St Laurence's Home for Catholic nurses was opened. The council of the Queen's Institute forwarded £140 to pay for the training of the first Catholic probationary nurses. Mrs Rathbone also promised £50 a year for four years if the home succeeded in receiving local support. In 1892, Miss Mansel, an inspector appointed by the council of the Queen's Institute, visited St Laurence's Home and expressed her satisfaction with the work being done there.[13]

By this time, one other training school, in addition to the two in Dublin, had been affiliated throughout Ireland – in Londonderry, established in 1891. Gradually the Queen's Institute began to receive applications for Queen's Nurses by local voluntarily organised committees throughout Ireland – the system of district nursing was beginning to spread across the country.

After its tenure in Mary Street, St Laurence's Home moved address when Lady O'Hagan offered the use of her house at 34 Rutland Square (now Parnell Square) to be used as the Catholic nurses' training home, at a rent of £1 per annum.[14] This house became the permanent headquarters for St Laurence's Home in affiliation with the Queen's Institute and remained a training home for nurses until its closure in 1953. It was a substantial house on the west side of Rutland Square, adjacent to the Rotunda Hospital. The home had as its patron Archbishop Walsh, with a general governing committee of over 40 members. At the first meeting of the friends and supporters of St Laurence's Home in November 1893, Archbishop Walsh, in his opening speech, highly praised the work of the Queen's Institute and the services of the district nurses. He commented that the home was worthy of public support and that the number of subscribers to it should be far in excess of the 70 subscribers it retained at that time, given that it serviced 35 parishes. He also mentioned the perception that St Laurence's Home was endowed and maintained by the Queen, which was completely wrong and which might have the effect of bringing the work of the home to a standstill. He praised Lady O'Hagan and the Earl of Meath for their generous work.[15]

The Irish branch of the Queen's Institute was now firmly established and the district nursing system was beginning to take root. However, it was going to take much local endeavour to establish district nursing associations that could afford and maintain a nurse for their own communities. By 1896 St Patrick's Home reported that there were 60 Queen's Nurses and associated district nursing associations affiliated with the Queen's Institute operating throughout Ireland.[16] Mr Harold Boulton, honorary treasurer of the Queen's Institute, commented at the time that 'no one imagined when the Queen first endowed the Charity how soon it would grow to the very large proportions it has now assumed. The demand for Queen's Nurses throughout the length and breadth of the land is far beyond our means of meeting it.'[17]

Queen Victoria died in January 1901 and was succeeded by her son Edward VII and his wife Princess Alexandra. Shortly thereafter William Rathbone died in March 1902. Both individuals had significant influence in the foundations of the district nursing system. The Rathbone family is still connected to the Queen's Nursing Institute in England but 'Old Rathbone', as Archbishop Walsh and Charles Kennedy referred to him in their communications, is one of the many people in Irish history who have unfortunately been forgotten.

VICEREGAL CONNECTION

The operation of the Irish branch of the Queen's Institute relied heavily on the participation and continued interest in the cause which was expressed by the wives of many of the viceroys to Ireland. As the Queen's representatives in Ireland, the position of the viceroy was very important. On 23 August 1899, *The Times* recorded that the presentation of badges and certificates to newly qualified district nurses took place the previous afternoon on the lawn in front of the Viceregal Lodge and was presided over by the viceroy's wife, Lady Cadogan.[18]

On the occasion of Queen Victoria's Diamond Jubilee in 1897, a large fund was raised by the people of Great Britain to support the Queen's Institute. Upon the Queen's death, a further fund of £84,600 was raised for the Women's Memorial to Queen Victoria. Of this fund, £6,000 was raised by a committee under the supervision of Lady Cadogan, and this portion of the fund was therefore allocated for use in Ireland.[19]

When Lord Dudley replaced Lord Cadogan in 1903, his wife Lady Rachel Dudley took a keen interest in district nursing and established Lady Dudley's Scheme which lasted until 1974. (This scheme is discussed in greater depth in Chapter 5.) Lady Dudley, whose husband was on very friendly terms with Edward VII and Princess Alexandra, was pivotal in her influence over the council of the Queen's Institute in convincing them to allocate the full £6,000 mentioned above for investment in her scheme, which amounted to £180 per annum.[20]

When Lord Aberdeen replaced Lord Dudley as viceroy in 1908, Lady Aberdeen immersed herself in Irish affairs, including the establishment of the Women's National Health Associations – local district nursing associations which were affiliated to the Queen's Institute (see Chapter 7).

THE IRISH ADVISORY COMMITTEE

In the early years of the Irish branch of the Queen's Institute, the organisation was administrated and funded by the Queen's Institute in London, under the supervision of an Irish Advisory Committee. The members of this committee were carefully nominated individuals who represented the elite of Irish society, encompassing landed gentry, wealthy merchants and loyal benefactors. These people continued to contribute voluntarily towards the work of the committee for many years and often into several generations.

It was the intention of the Queen's Institute in London that Wales and Ireland should operate under their own separate council to delegate responsibility for operations to each individual territory. Mary Lamont, superintendent of the Queen's Institute in Ireland from 1898 to 1912, opened discussion for the establishment of a separate Irish Executive Committee based in Dublin. Lamont's work covered a broad range of activities, and she felt that the establishment of an Executive Committee in Dublin would reduce the need to report back to the Council of the Queen's Institute in London on such a regular basis in exchange for funding. Unfortunately for Mary Lamont, this proposal was not accepted

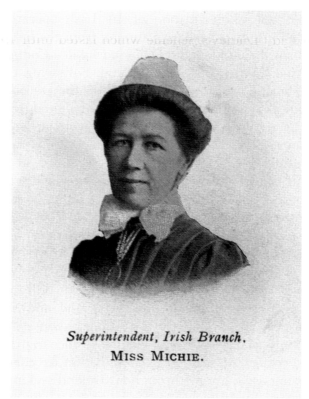

Superintendent, Irish Branch.
MISS MICHIE.

Miss Michie, Superintendent, Irish Branch 1912–1928. Courtesy of Queen's Nursing Institute, London.

by the Irish Advisory Committee and local district nursing associations who were happy to continue with the status quo and to receive funding from London, despite the immense administrative effort and inconvenience placed on the superintendent.

Mary Lamont resigned after thirteen years and was succeeded in 1912 by Annie Michie. Upon the coming into being of the Irish Free State in 1922, the Irish Advisory Committee became the Irish Executive Committee, in line with new political structures in the country and reflective of the original proposal by Mary Lamont.

FUNDRAISING UNDER THE IRISH FREE STATE

The financial administration of the Queen's Institute in Ireland changed with the introduction of the Irish Free State and the Irish Executive Committee in 1922. The Queen's Institute had previously funded the administration of its Irish operations, which amounted to roughly £2,000 per annum, from the balance of the dividends from the Golden and Diamond Jubilee Commemoration Funds and the Women's Memorial Fund. Following the declaration of the Irish Free State, the council of the Queen's Institute did not think it equitable to use money contributed by the people of England and Wales for the support of work in Ireland.[21] The subsidy granted from central funds of the Queen's Institute was reduced in gradual stages. In 1923 this was £1,000; in 1924 it was £600; and in 1925 it was reduced to £400 after which the subsidy was discontinued except for the grant of £100 from the Queen from the proceeds of Alexandra Day.[22]

Funding the general operation of the Irish branch of the Queen's Institute was now the responsibility of the Irish Executive Committee and was going to require a capital fund of at least £40,000 to extend their work in Ireland. Expenditure consisted of special district training for the nurses and midwifery where required; inspection of districts; travelling expenses; salaries of superintendents and inspectors; lectures; office rent; and print and postage costs.[23] Accordingly, the affiliation fee charged to the district nursing associations throughout Ireland seeking affiliation with the Queen's Institute was increased to £2.2.0 for single-nurse associations, with a further 10s 6d for each additional nurse on staff.

The Irish Executive Committee was also now responsible for raising its own endowment fund for the nurses' pensions. This was because most district nursing associations were barely able to pay everyday salary and expenses for their existing nurse and were not in a position to pay for her comfortable retirement. Queen's nurses were encouraged to remain single and to devote their lives, and in many cases health, to the community. From very early in the Institute's history it was realised that a special fund would have to be set up to take proper care of retired nurses. The Countess of Kenmare spoke of this, as president in 1929, in the foreword of the Annual Report of the Queen's Institute.

> It is not much to ask that when our nurses can no longer face the daily round, the far from common task, we, who stand by admiring and respectful, should remember that we must yield something more substantial than admiration and respect if we are to make their future safe.[24]

Many of the later appeals and fundraising events were for pensions for retired nurses. It became a greater preoccupation because of the numbers of nurses retired. The first annuities from this fund were paid to Queen's Nurses in July 1930. By 31 December of that year there were thirteen nurses on the pension roll and the conditions of eligibility were that a Queen's Nurse must be at least 55 years of age, have completed 21 years' service and must have resigned from district nursing. The amount given to each retired nurse was £30 per annum, paid quarterly.[25]

Fundraising began in earnest throughout the country in every town and village where there was a Queen's Nurse in service, and much of what was donated and collected went specifically towards the nurses' pension fund. There were flag days, bridge tournaments, golf tournaments, tennis tournaments, whist drives, dog shows and even a rodeo.[26] These were organised by the committees of the district nursing associations and supported by a network of loyal subscribers and collectors located throughout Ireland and Great Britain. Contributors to this fund were thanked every year for their generosity to nursing associations who found themselves in financial difficulty. One such organisation was the Irish Peasant Society in London. They contributed annually to most of the District

Nursing Associations as well as directly to the Irish branch of the Queen's Institute of District Nursing, both North and South.[27]

GARDEN SCHEME

When asked about their memories of Jubilee nurses, many people will say it reminds them of tea in beautiful gardens, and they often do not know why this is. It may be because of the very successful garden scheme that was devised in 1926 by Ms Elsie Wagg of the Council of the Queen's Institute in England. It still operates as the National Gardens Scheme in Britain, raising funds for several charitable organisations including the Queen's Institute. Garden owners allowed the public to view their gardens for a small fee. In many areas where there was an active district nursing association or particularly enthusiastic owner, tea or light refreshments were offered as part of the entry fee. Mrs Barry of Ongar, Clonsilla, Dublin initiated the scheme in Ireland in 1929 and worked towards its realisation as a countrywide fundraiser. In 1930, 311 gardens were opened, and in excess of £4,000 was raised. The funds were divided equally between the local district nursing association and the pension fund administered by the Queen's Institute in Dublin.

It was an opportunity for the owners of some of the most spectacular gardens in the country to show them at their most beautiful. The numbers of gardens opened would indicate that many gardens of different merits were displayed. A large committee was formed with membership – and secretary – in almost every county in Ireland. The list of this committee in 1930 is interesting because the members came from some of the most beautiful gardens now open to the public today. This list includes, among many others, the Honourable Mrs Plunkett of St Anne's, Clontarf, Dublin, Mr Horace Walpole of Mount Usher, Wicklow, Mrs Edmund Darley of Fern Hill, Sandyford, County Dublin, and Mrs Leigh-White of Bantry House, County Cork. Writing in the *Irish Times* in May 1956 Miss Sheila Pim spoke of some of the ten new gardens that had been opened in the scheme that year. 'Most, though not all, of the gardens are on the grand scale. Their attractions vary from forestry and bluebell woods, as on the Viscount De Vesci's estate in Leix, to small rare rock plants. Among those soon to be on view are several famous for rhododendrons, Howth Castle, and the Countess of Leitrim's fine collection at Mulroy, Co. Donegal.'[28] Many of the most successful open garden days were in the Dublin area. In 1935 £778. 2/- 11d was raised despite the Tramway and bus strike in Dublin which lasted for eleven weeks disrupting spring and summer viewings.[29] During the 1940s 'Emergency' it was not always possible to organise the garden scheme due to petrol shortages and tea rationing.[30] These difficulties were overcome and the scheme continued to enhance the pension fund for retired nurses long after the Queen's Institute had ceased general operations.

NEW COUNCIL OF THE QUEEN'S INSTITUTE, IRISH BRANCH – 1930s

In 1930 the Queen's Institute, Irish branch was reorganised. A council governing all of Ireland was created by incorporating the Executive Committee of the Irish Free State and the Executive Committee of Northern Ireland. This central council was made up of representatives of both of these committees as well as representatives from St Patrick's Home and St Laurence's Home, under the presidency of the Countess of Kenmare. The total number of local district nursing associations was 123 in the Irish Free State and 35 in Northern Ireland. The two Executive Committees on either side of the border were to operate independently of one another but would be accountable to the Central Council governing all of Ireland.

In 1933, the *Irish Times* reported on the importance of the Queen's Institute in Ireland as representing a cross-border organisation which aimed to serve all, regardless of political and religious belief, in line with the original ethos represented by William Rathbone on its establishment in Ireland in the late 1800s. 'The Institute is one of those few bodies which still preserves the reality of a united Ireland. Its influence radiates into every county, its workers possess the respect and love of all classes. The organisation soars above politics, as it soars above partition.'[31]

In Northern Ireland, the local authorities took over financial responsibility of the entire home nursing service under the National Health Scheme on 5 July 1948. The local committees of the district nursing associations were disbanded, the Belfast office of the Northern Ireland Executive Committee was closed, and the inspector for Northern Ireland found her post redundant.[32] Miss Colburn, superintendent of the Institute, wrote to the local district nursing associations explaining that:

> The Northern Ireland nurses have not been given notice. Every nurse has been taken over by the County Medical Officer of Health. The local Committees have been asked to continue to take an interest in the work of the nurse and provide additional comforts for the patients. The only change is that the local committees are relieved of all financial responsibility, as the nurses' salaries and all expenses will be paid by the County Authorities, under the new National Health Insurance Bill.[33]

A new Constitution and Rules of the Queen's Institute in Ireland was drafted in 1950 which redefined the aims and objective of the organisation as the training and provision of district nurses and the supervision of these nurses and their district nursing associations. This constitution also defined the new structure of the central council which was to consist of not less than 21 and not more than 27 members, made up of individuals representing a broad spectrum of Irish society.

THE WAR YEARS

The years between 1939 and 1945 marked a state-declared 'emergency' within Ireland, due to the impact of the Second World War throughout Europe. The operation of the Queen's Institute and its district nursing associations in Ireland was just as significantly impacted as any other body at that time. All fundraising efforts suffered during this period, and a shortage of petrol forced the Queen's Institute to immobilise the three motor cars provided for the superintendent and inspectors, who were instead provided with bicycles and often covered 30 to 40 miles a day. During the war, and primarily between October 1940 and June 1941, the Jubilee nurses, together with their superintendent, received and cared for over 2,000 refugee infants and small children who arrived into Dún Laoghaire in Dublin by mail boat every evening. This year also saw the first broadcast appeal for funds from Radio Éireann by the superintendent of the Queen's Institute in Ireland, which generated donations from Scotland, England, Northern Ireland and the Republic of Ireland.[34]

THE DEMISE OF THE QUEEN'S INSTITUTE

The reasons for the demise of the Queen's Institute and its affiliated organisations are very complex. As discussed earlier, there was an overall aspiration in 1947 within changing governments of the Irish state to provide community services from the public purse. That said, they were very happy with the continued provision of a service by the Queen's Institute which they themselves were not in a position to provide at the time. This contradiction between statements and actions created much difficulty for the Queen's Institute towards the end of the scheme. In 1953 the service provided by the Institute was still perceived by the Department of Health as a 'cheap' yet more efficient means of providing domiciliary nursing care. A ten-page interdepartmental letter sent in 1953 regarding 'outdoor services' – or community care services – to the Department of Finance ends with:

> The Minister might, therefore, be subject to some criticism for supporting from public monies an organisation whose controlling body is not democratically elected and the constitution of which the hospitals commission described as 'perpetuating a suggestion of external control'. Since however, local authorities would be doing no more than using the associations to supply them with nurses, it can be maintained that there is no need to upset the 'flavour' attaching to them, and that the minister would be no more vulnerable on this score than he would because he allows local authorities to make use of, say, some of the voluntary hospitals whose governing bodies would be open to the same objection.[35]

As mentioned above, the operation of the Irish branch of the Queen's Institute was completely independent of English control. The 'flavour' mentioned in the letter describes the perception that both the Queen's Institute and district nursing associations were Protestant in character. However, the Queen's Institute was constituted with a strong non-denominational ethos and, as will be demonstrated in further discussion of the district nursing associations, there was no pattern of religious bias at all. While there were many government meetings, often instigated by the Queen's Institute, there was obviously no attempt made to understand the true composition of the associations or the extent of the valuable contribution they were making to the economy or society as a whole.

In 1966 another white paper was drafted on the health services. A circular on district nursing services was sent to all voluntary nursing services. This circular set out very carefully that the 'fullest use should, of course, continue to be made of the services of district nurses employed by voluntary nursing agencies in the organisation of community health services'.[36] This was the year before the Queen's Institute training school was indirectly closed by An Bord Altranais, the state body responsible for regulating the standards of nursing training in Ireland which was established in 1950. One of the misgivings that the Queen's Institute had about this circular was that 'in view of a long practical experience in the field of district nursing they were not given the opportunity of offering their views on how the further expansion of the domiciliary nursing services could be best achieved'.

Criticism of the perceived ethos of the Queen's Institute by the government was counterbalanced by increasing subventions of finance to district nursing associations by local government authorities. In 1956 the local authorities were given permission to increase funding to up to 75 per cent of the district nursing association's costs. Grants were only offered to district nursing associations, at the discretion of the County Manager, when evidence of reasonable efforts to raise funds locally was presented by the secretary of the association. The amount of financial support for some districts varied and remained confidential despite the reality that most nursing associations were providing a similar service. Later this figure increased to 85 per cent of costs. It was, however, still dependent on the application for funding by the secretary of each district nursing association.[37]

A difficulty encountered by the Queen's Institute in the 1960s was that the Irish Nurses Organisation (INO) (a union representing most nurses qualified and in training) had been concerned for some time that conditions for Queen's nurses were not of the same standard as those for district nurses in state employment. In 1965 the INO questioned the Institute regarding pensions for married nurses, some of whom had contributed a very long service in a temporary capacity.[38] The INO was vocal in its insistence on equal pay for nurses in public and private services and also for suitable pension arrangements in both. District nursing associations were struggling to provide an adequate salary for their nurses. This was often due to a lack of interest among the general public because public health nurses were available in other districts and did not require the fundraising efforts of the public in order to function.

The ultimate reason for the closure of the Queen's Institute was the shortage of probationary nurses to train and place in districts. In 1955 proposals were formulated by An Bord Altranais to introduce postgraduate training of nurses for domiciliary work. In a memo circulated in 1956, the Minister for Health, Thomas O'Higgins, reassured the Queen's Institute that their training homes would continue regardless of whether the proposals of An Bord Altranais were adopted or not.[39] In a letter to the secretary of the Department of Health in 1963, the Queen's Institute suggested that, in cooperation with An Bord Altranais, a combined course for public health and district nursing of six months should be introduced.[40] A 1966 brief to the new Minister for Health, Seán Flanagan, outlined the discussions between An Bord Altranais and the Queen's Institute regarding the training of Jubilee nurses and informed him that they were trying to reach agreement on a coordinated course but had failed to do so. An Bord Altranais went ahead and organised their training course. This action led to the establishment of a separate public health nurse qualification. The brief to the minister continued: 'An Bord are not prepared to recognize the Jubilee Training for qualification and the Institute do not regard this as satisfactory.'[41] Nurses who were trained by and working for the Queen's Institute were no longer registered or permitted to work for state agencies without further qualifications. Following the introduction of this Public Health Training Course by An Bord Altranais, applications for the Queen's Institute training course rapidly declined. The new course offered candidates better working conditions and permanence of employment on qualification. The training homes had been doomed from the inception of An Bord Altranais despite earlier assurance by the government. Throughout this unsettled period of negotiations with the government, the Queen's Institute was in communication with no less than thirteen Ministers for Health.

In 1953, St Laurence's Training Home was closed and three years later, St Patrick's Training Home relocated to Morehampton Road, Dublin 4, where it continued to operate as a training home and base for district nursing services provided to the people of the local community for several years. On 30 June 1968, however, the Queen's Institute of District Nursing ceased its training

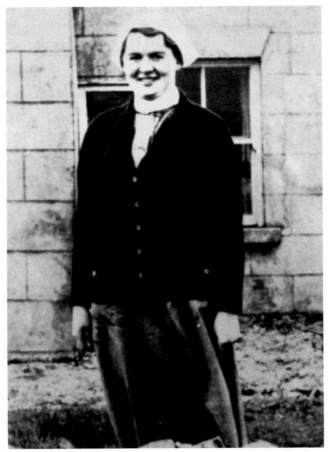

Miss Mary Quain, the last superintendent of the Queen's Institute in Ireland. Photographed during her time as a Lady Dudley's nurse in Carraroe, County Galway. Courtesy of Kenny's Bookshop, County Galway.

activities after nearly 75 years. In September 1968 Mary Quain, the last superintendent of the Queen's Institute in Ireland, wrote to all district nursing associations calling an extraordinary general meeting, the result of which was the closure of the Queen's Institute. Several district nursing associations continued to operate but eventually closed when their nurse retired or left for other reasons. The Institute continued the administration of the pension fund and in 2003 the Trust Funds of the Queen's Institute of District Nursing were amalgamated into one fund by a cy-près order of the Commissioners for Charitable Donations and Bequests.[42]

ACKNOWLEDGEMENTS

During the 1940s several of the founding members of the Queen's Institute passed away.

Elizabeth the Countess of Kenmare, first President of the Council for all of Ireland (born 1867), who established one of the first district nursing associations in 1899, which was based in Killarney, died in 1944. In her memory Lt Col McGillycuddy of the Reeks organised an appeal for funds to augment the nurses' pension fund which was established by the countess in 1927. Geraldine Countess of Mayo (born 1863) also died in 1944. The countess assisted Lady Dudley in her foundation and maintenance of Lady Dudley's Scheme. The Honourable Mrs Florence Barry, founder of the Garden Scheme and a long-serving member of the Council of the Queen's Institute in Ireland, died in 1941. Many of the members of the Council and Committees of the Queen's Institute voluntarily gave lifelong dedication to the cause of the provision of district nursing services throughout the country over many decades. It could not be possible to record every person who made such a commitment throughout Ireland over such a long period of time because the numbers are so large, but they should be acknowledged for their immense contribution and commendable effort.

A letter of thanks from the Queen Mother was received by the Queen's Institute in Ireland on 6 June 1968.[43]

CONTEMPORARY CORRESPONDENCE AROUND THE TIME THAT THE IRISH QUEEN'S INSTITUTE WAS SET UP

Lady Aberdeen, who was wife of the viceroy to Ireland in 1886, wrote to Archbishop Walsh in Dublin in 1889, at a particularly difficult time when there was no agreement on the provision of training for Catholic nurses. She had only just become a member of the Council for Queen's Institute in Scotland that year. The letter highlights the deep commitment of Lady Aberdeen and her desire to use all her contacts for the good of the organisation.

27 Grosvenor Square W.

March 25th 1889

My dear Archbishop,

I have to thank your Grace for your kind letter of the 10th. I am much obliged to you for writing and telling me the reasons of the failure of the Queen's Jubilee Nursing Institute in Ireland. I will try in some way or another to let her Majesty know how it is that it has failed, but you will understand that it is not a very easy matter for me and I must think how it can best be done. I cannot say that I am surprised at the result.

We have at last settled in our new house here and we hope very much that you will be coming over during the season and that we may have the pleasure of seeing your Grace here and talking over many matters which are full of interest to us.

With Lord Aberdeen's kindest regards.

Believe me,
yours very sincerely,
Ishbel Aberdeen[44]

In the next letter, from Florence Nightingale to Mr Rathbone, the influential Miss Nightingale was also concerned, at that time, about the serious difficulties everyone had trying to set up the voluntary district nursing scheme that was so desperately needed in Ireland.

PRIVATE May 13/89
10, South Street
Park Lane
Q.V.J.I.N

Dear Mr Rathbone,

For your valuable documents I have most carefully read and pondered, namely

Sir R. Alcock's 'Note' on 'Dublin Nursing Assoc'

Your Memo on this 'Note'

Mr Bonham Carter's Letters to you of May 1

Your Memo on that letter

As you are so good as to wish me to say something, I can only say what you do not wish me to say, that your boundless generosity is so deeply felt in regard to this your scheme, meaning the District Nursing plan of Superintendent and Nurses drawn from the three Institutions.

And it is so well understood how desirable it is for the sake of Ireland now to take advantage of it that one can only bid you God speed amidst difficulties which are enormous, but which, as you so justly say, are opportunities for who knows how to profit by them.

Under the circumstances it may well be that there is no alternative and I need hardly assure you that our best wishes are yours that it may succeed in the highest sense. Let everyone concerned endeavor [sic] to work out your proposals in the same spirit as yourself; and that <u>will</u> be success.

I would say; We pray God that it may succeed. But we know already that He wishes wishes [sic] the greatest good to this Nursing of His sick poor, even more than we can. In Him therefore who inspires you we put our trust. May he give many more years of you to this kingdom.

Every yours gratefully & truly

Florence Nightingale
I always send you my gratitude in my heart for all your kindness to me. May I add this now in ink? F.N.[45]

Mr Rathbone and Mr Henry Tate both made large donations to the fund. Mr Tate made a donation in the amount of £5,000 together with a letter stipulating exactly how he would like this money to be used.

NOTES

1 Notice in *The Times*, December 1887, SA/QNI/S2/1, Box 120. The Queen's Nursing Institute (hereafter QNI) Archives, Wellcome Library, London.

2 Queen Victoria's Jubilee Institute for Nurses (hereafter QVJIN), Charter of Incorporation, September 1889, p. 2. The Queen's Nursing Institute, London.

3 QVJIN Regulations, Final Meeting of Provisional Committee, February 1890, p. xi, SA/QNI/S2/1, Box 120. QNI Archives, Wellcome Library, London.

4 St Patrick's Home, 13th Annual Report, 1889, p. 8. National Archives, Dublin.

5 Ibid.

6 *Queen's Nurses' Magazine* (1905), p. 101. The Queen's Nursing Institute, London.

7 Minutes of Provisional Committee, July 1888, SA/QNI/C.1/1–2. QNI Archives, Wellcome Library, London.

8 St Patrick's Home, 13th Annual Report, 1889, p. 4. National Archives, Dublin.

9 Minutes of Governing Body and Letters from Committee, SA/QNI/ S2/1/1, Box 120. QNI Archives, Wellcome Library, London.

10 Letter from Miss Dunn to Colonel Gildea, 3 June 1890. SA/QNI/S2/1/1, Box 120. QNI Archives, Wellcome Library, London.

11 Minutes of QVJIN 7th Meeting, December 1890, p. 43. The Queen's Nursing Institute, London.

12 Minutes of Sub-Committee Meeting, 3 March 1890, SA/QNI/S2/1/1–2, QNI Archives, Wellcome Library, London.

13 QVJIN Dublin Affiliation Meeting, *Irish Times*, 11 June 1892, p. 6. Irish Times Archives.

14 St Laurence's Catholic Home, 3rd Annual Report, December 1894. *Irish Times*, 7 December 1894, p. 6. Irish Times Archives.

15 Archbishop Walsh, St Laurence's Catholic Home, Annual Meeting, 20 November 1893, Speech, pp. 18–22, SA/QNI/C.5/2. QNI Archives, Wellcome Library, London.

16 St Patrick's Home, Annual Report, 1896, p. 15. National Archives Dublin.

17 St Patrick's Home, Annual Report, 1901, p. 10. National Archives Dublin.

18 *Irish Times*, 23 August 1899. Irish Times Archives.

19 QVJIN Women's Memorial Committee Report, December 1903. The Queen's Nursing Institute, London.

20   QVJIN Council Minutes 1903. SA/QNI/C.1/1–2. QNI Archives, Wellcome Library, London.

21   QVJIN Irish Branch, 1st Annual Report, 1924, p. 4. National Archives, Dublin.

22   QVJIN, Annual Report 1923, Report of Council to Patron Queen Alexandra, p. 23. The Queen's Nursing Institute, London.

23   QVJIN Irish Branch, 1st Annual Report, 1924, p. 8. National Archives, Dublin.

24   Lady Kenmare, President, Queen's Institute of District Nurses (hereafter QIDN) Irish Branch Annual Report, 1928, Foreword, p. 12. National Archives, Dublin.

25   QIDN Irish Branch, 1st Annual Report of New Council, 1930, p. 12. National Archives, Dublin.

26   QVJIN Irish Branch, 1st Annual Report, 1924, p. 26. National Archives, Dublin.

27   This is recorded in nearly every Annual Report.

28   Miss Sheila Pim, 'Open for Charity', Irish Times, 12 May 1956, p. 8. Irish Times Archives.

29   QIDN Annual Report, 1935, p. 10, QI DN1, Box 23. National Archives, Dublin.

30   QIDN Annual Report, 1941, p. 5, QI DN1, Box 23. National Archives, Dublin.

31   QIDN Report of AGM, Irish Times, 17 March 1933, p. 6. Irish Times Archives.

32   QIDN, Report of Executive Committee of Éire, 31 December 1948, p. 4. National Archives, Dublin.

33   Letter from Miss Colburn to Mrs Poole, Cahir DNA, 3 May 1948. Inventory No. 1991.186. South Tipperary County Museum.

34   QIDN, Report of Executive Committee of Éire, 31 December 1941, p. 5. National Archives, Dublin.

35   Department of Health files, M100/150. National Archives, Dublin.

36   Circular 27/66 from Department of Health, Department of Health files, M/15/13. National Archives, Dublin

37   Letter to City/County Manager, 5 Samhain 1956, Department of Health files, M27/13. National Archives, Dublin.

38   Irish Nurses' Organisation Annual Report, 1965, Department of Health files, M100/150. National Archives, Dublin.

39   Memo, 20 Iúil 1956, Department of Health files, M100/259/vol. 2. National Archives, Dublin.

40   Letter from QIDN to Secretary, Department of Health, 29 November 1963, Department of Health files, M115/13, M28/5. National Archives, Dublin.

41   Deputation from QIDN, Brief for Minister, 13 December 1966, Department of Health files, M115/13. National Archives, Dublin.

42   Commissioners of Charitable Donations and Bequests for Ireland, Cy-Pres
       Scheme, March 2003. The Queen's Nursing Institute, London.
43   Copy of letter of acknowledgement to letter of thanks from Her Majesty
       Queen Elizabeth The Queen Mother, 17 July 1968. The Queen's Nursing
       Institute, London.
44   Letter from Lady Aberdeen to Archbishop Walsh, March 1889, Archbishop
       Walsh Papers, Archbishop's Palace, Dublin.
45   Letter from Florence Nightingale to Mr Rathbone, May 1889, SA/QNI/
       S2/1 Box 120. QNI Archives, Wellcome Library, London.

CHAPTER 3

District Nursing Associations

Ramelton District Nursing Fund

FANCY FAIR & SALE

IN THE

TOWN HALL, RAMELTON

——: ON :——

Wednesday, 27th Nov.

There will be numerous Stalls, including Work, Farm Produce, Cake and Jelly.

TEAS and REFRESHMENTS

—— A SPECIALITY. ——

SIDE :: SHOWS

Including Shooting, Palmistry, &c.

The Sale will be opened at 3 o'clock by Lady STEWART.

Admission : : Fourpence

Proceeds in aid of above Fund.

ALL ARE HEARTILY INVITED

Printed by W. Barr & Son, Letterkenny.

Courtesy of Copyright Donegal County Archives, P27.

During the presence of the Queen's Institute in Ireland, 327 district nursing associations (DNAs) were established and scattered throughout the country in the first half of the twentieth century.[1] These associations were a perfect example of social capital working at its most efficient and effective. The core function of these associations was to provide a domiciliary nursing service for its local town or village. Each had a unique character reflecting that of the people involved in their management and, in many instances, the Jubilee nurse, who often remained in the district of the association for many years. Committees were formed to run these associations and interested participants gathered together and pledged time, energy and often social reputation to the cause. A leading member of the community – who may have been the parish priest or other clergy, doctor, local landowner or businessperson – would usually act as the head of a committee. If the committee decided that it would be appropriate to commission a nurse to work among the poor of the parish, an application for such a nurse was made to the Queen's Institute. Upon the granting of a nurse, the association was then affiliated with the Institute. These associations, and the Jubilee nurses provided to them, gave each town a strong bond of social cohesion as the community had to work together to fund the nurse, not just occasionally but repeatedly and over many decades. Each district would often have hundreds of members subscribing to the local district nursing association on a yearly basis. The administration of these fundraising efforts was carried out by the committee, who met monthly and who recruited volunteers to work for the cause.

The first district nursing association affiliated in Ireland was Omagh District Nursing Association in 1891. The last committee was set up in 1958 (affiliated in 1960) in Walkinstown, Dublin. The total number of affiliated district nursing associations includes the committee of Lady Dudley's Scheme. The service offered by Lady Dudley's Scheme was effectively that offered by a large district nursing association.

The list of affiliated branches begins with a description of the establishment of each district nursing association. It always named the honorary secretary and, in later decades, the entire committee is named. They describe the nurse's accommodation and salary and any other factors pertinent to living conditions which were offered by the association to their nurse. It records whether midwifery was to be practised in the district and whether patients' fees were to be charged. Each district nursing association also had to calculate the approximate population the nurse would be responsible for. This was important as it was necessary to have a sufficiently strong financial base to support the nurse. It was also necessary to ensure that the population would be manageable by one – albeit highly efficient – district nurse. Sometimes a large population would demand that two nurses be employed. Changes in these initial records were updated, but not very consistently, by the superintendent for the Queen's Institute. Changes were made to the lists according to the findings of annual inspections regarding affiliations, disaffiliations and the transfer of nurses.

The geographical spread of district nursing associations was not uniform throughout the country. The figure above included district nursing associations for the North of Ireland until 1929. The Irish branch and Northern Ireland branch of the Queen's Institute divided into two councils that year. The Irish branch did not record district nursing associations in the North of Ireland after this date.[2]

All of the larger towns had a jubilee nurse, or two, but there were many counties where only a limited number of towns or villages had a nurse. County Donegal was exceptional with 40 voluntary nursing associations, many of which were set up in the 1930s. Some were part of Lady Dudley's Scheme, several were traditional district nursing associations, three were part of the McDevitt Nursing Scheme (a charitable bequest that subsidised nurses in the Glenties area) and several were referred to as 'health clubs'. Health clubs were conceived by Dr Seán Ó Deagha (O'Dea), the first County Medical Officer of Health in Donegal in the early 1930s. The idea was, according to Dr Ó Deagha, to 'interest the general public; to have at least one member of every household in the district belong to the club, and so to obviate, to some extent, the difficulty which is being generally experienced at the present time of collecting subscriptions'.[3] These health clubs tended to have a parish priest as president.

THE COMMITTEE

Committees tended to be composed of a classic stereotype of members – they were people with the time and the financial means to support the work. In the early years, district nursing associations were likely to have a predominantly female committee; the president was often a titled lady. Committees met once a month and more frequently when an event was being organised. The importance of a supportive committee to the work of the nurse was regularly noted in the annual reports of the Queen's Institute.[4] The necessity for good communication between nurses and their committee was implicit, and was also formalised, by the requirement for nurses to give a monthly report to their committee. This report assisted all parties in maintaining a positive relationship and constantly reinforced the motivation for their work. Miss Aylward, Superintendent for Ireland, speaking to a world congress of nurses in Quebec, Canada in 1954 stated: 'It is most important that the committee members be kept interested in the work of the association, they receive from Nurse reports of work done, in writing and verbally, without in any way violating the confidence of the patients.'[5]

In the 1930s, many of the committees formed to run district nursing associations were made up entirely of female members, but towards the end of that decade the composition of the committees began to take a different flavour with the local parish priest often becoming president to a female honorary secretary – often a school teacher – and the local bank manager or his wife acting as honorary treasurer.

In order to operate efficiently, district nursing associations had a large core of regularly contributing members and subscribers. The number of ordinary members depended on the structure of the association and the size of the town. As well as providing subscriptions, ordinary members were the foot soldiers to help in the arduous but often enjoyable task of raising funds to provide a salary, keep, transport and pension for the nurse. Committees usually drew as their participants the more enthusiastic ordinary members. Nurses and members came and went but what endured over many decades was the ethos and commitment to continue the work for the benefit of the community.

The honourable secretary of the committee was usually a woman. In 1935, of the 170 district nursing associations in the country, fifteen men were appointed as secretaries. Of these, four were religious pastors, three were parish priests, and one was a rector. Many of the other men on the list appear to have addresses in schools or estate offices.[6] The job required a considerable time commitment and organisational ability. The secretary was usually the person responsible for the supervision and assistance of the nurses in the day-to-day management of their work and accommodation. The success – or failure – of a district nursing association was usually dependent on the person chosen to be secretary of the committee. A succession of strong women in the position of honorary secretary was the common denominator through all of the districts studied in detail. Birr District Nursing Association, for example, was blessed in having, in its 66 years running, three very efficient secretaries who were kept in check by two generations of Lady Ross acting as president. The district had many nurses but the strength of the association lay in the committee itself.

THE PROVISION OF A JUBILEE NURSE

Most of the large towns had at least one nurse and there was often competition for nurses between communities. The *Queen's Nurses' Magazine* reported on the annual general meeting of the Cork District Nursing Association in May 1906. It came as a surprise to the members that Cork city had only one nurse while Londonderry, a smaller city, had five.[7] The Cork District Nursing Association was in existence from 1900 until 1966 but never employed more than one nurse at a time. This example shows the very patchy nature of the provision of voluntary district nurses in Ireland. The *Sligo Champion* of 31 October 1936 discussed the high rate of child mortality, which could have been avoided if another nurse was in the town. The reporter believed that other towns of a similar size had at least three nurses.[8] However, the provision of a second nurse was a decision that was not taken lightly by a committee and was scrutinised by the Queen's Institute very thoroughly before permission was granted. Some areas had a strong committee and sufficient local support and were able to provide more than one nurse. In later decades, and as populations increased, local government subventions were given to associations to support a second nurse.

The professional longevity of the nurse in many parishes dictated the permanence of the association itself. Many folded when a nurse retired or was married. Districts often stayed open until the nurse was ready to retire.

In some districts that remained open for a long period, this longevity could be attributed not to one but two or three nurses. Often, upon establishment of an association, a good nurse could help to stabilise the committee and its work. Towards the end, when financial difficulties crushed many associations, a strong Jubilee nurse could sustain the work.

Transfers of nurses within the network of districts were regularly arranged by the Queen's Institute, although they did not follow any pattern or rationale. Sometimes the transfer was executed in order to assist the nurse to find a district with which she was compatible. This flexibility was an advantage for the Queen's Institute, which needed to replace nurses who required leave of absence for indefinite periods, usually due to illness or to assist in 'home duties' – an elderly or dying parent. The Institute trained and regularly reviewed the nurse and, as a result, would have had good knowledge of all her capabilities. District nursing associations were generally happier to receive a nurse who had some experience. Lady Dudley's districts were not given a choice. The committees with a good working relationship with the Queen's Institute naturally had a better chance of acquiring a good nurse. Exceptional nurses were taken back to the training homes in Dublin and Londonderry to supervise students on the district. Usually nurses viewed life in urban or small towns as more comfortable than in the wilds of the west of Ireland and were only too happy to move. In many cases, temporary transfers became permanent.

The Lady Dudley's Scheme began a policy, a few years after it was established, which limited nurses' stay in each district to not more than three years due to the great isolation of these rural areas.[9] As a result, some of these districts seem to have been used as a sort of internship or introduction to district nursing. For example, Carna district in Galway began in 1903 and closed in 1967 and employed

30 nurses during its existence. The high turnover of nurses during this period indicates that very few had to endure significant time in these remote districts.

Marriage was the largest cause of loss of nurses to the districts as it was not possible for a nurse to continue to work after marriage. Some districts seem to have been particularly unlucky in this regard, such as Carlow District Nursing Association which lost six nurses to marriage between the years 1909 and 1966. Many districts simply closed on the marriage of the nurse. The life-style of the Jubilee nurse was not seen as compatible with family life as the nurse was effectively on call all of the time, except for one month of holidays every year. In later years, a solution was provided by the re-acceptance of married nurses back into their roles, albeit on a temporary basis. The reality of the situation, however, was that there was nothing temporary about these roles – many married women worked in a 'temporary' capacity for many decades. Regardless of her length of service, a Jubilee nurse who was married was never entitled to a pension upon retirement.

The reason nurses left their districts varied periodically. For some it was due to ill health, an occupational hazard for the Jubilee nurses, while waves of emigration took others to Canada, the US or to unspecified destinations. Many districts lost their nurse during the Great War on active service, while the Second World War also claimed some of the jubilee nurses when they joined the United Nations Relief and Rehabilitation Administration (UNRRA).[10] Several districts were reported to have lost nurses because they entered convents.

As working conditions improved for the public health nurses, many more Jubilee nurses left their associations to work for the government, often within the same, or neighbouring, communities where they had previously worked under the Queen's Institute. They were keen to leave their positions as Jubilee nurses in order to avoid round-the-clock duty calls, with only a half day off a week and one month's leave a year. This had been the norm for many years but it had become an out-of-date system and could not be sustained. The departure of nurses began slowly but was wide-spread by the 1960s when the local district nursing associations began to encounter difficulties raising funds and nurses began to recognise this threat to their posts. The committees struggled not just with finances but with old-fashioned ideologies. The ethos that had developed in many voluntary associations was in sympathy with Dr Coey Bigger's notion in 1920 that the ladies of the committee should be directly involved with the nurse's work. He said in a lecture that 'Ladies of the district could look after and help the nurses, and go with the nurse and take an interest in the cases, and so on, and in that way help the nurses to get in touch with every case of illness'.[11] Dr Coey Bigger was highly influential in the provision of all medical services in Ireland before and shortly after the formation of the Irish Free State. He was a council member of the Queen's Institute for many years. The nurses respected the suggestions of the doctor, and even those of some of the clergy, and took them on board when visiting the patients of the district.

The nurses respected the suggestions of the doctor, and even some of the clergy, when out and about visiting the patients of the district. Tensions often resulted from the necessity of the nurse to report to the committee and yet to keep them at a professional distance. As leading members of the community, paying the nurses' salary, the ladies of the committee were used to being in control of everything. They were aware of the necessity for patient confidentiality and yet human nature would have overcome this necessary discipline from time to time. A later nurse described the president of the district nursing association, with no medical training, on horseback checking 'whether the nurse had called to the cottages'. To a professional, highly trained nurse this seemed more than a little arrogant.[12] Mediating between all of the different parties in a district may have been an unacknowledged skill that nurses had to develop.

MIDWIFERY

Not all Jubilee nurses practised midwifery, but all who did were furnished with the necessary qualifications. It was up to the district nursing association to decide whether midwifery was to be offered to the people. Local authority grants were available to the district nursing association if they offered midwifery. As in the case of the dispensary doctors, there was an attempt to provide midwives throughout the whole country particularly after the 1917 Midwives (Ireland) Act. This legislation was an attempt to prevent unqualified 'handy women' from delivering babies. By 1920 most dispensary districts had a qualified midwife of some sort.[13] In 1935, of the 170 Queen's Institute districts, only 72 affiliated district nursing associations offered midwifery. Most of those were in Lady Dudley's Scheme, but, for instance, the nurse in Cappoquin District Nursing Association in Waterford delivered 37 babies that year.[14]

RELATIONSHIP WITH THE QUEEN'S INSTITUTE

The main function of the Queen's Institute in their engagement with local district nursing associations was the training, appointment and care of the nurses which the associations applied for and supervised. As a result, members of the Institute also found themselves becoming mentors and supervisors of vast numbers of voluntary lay people. The committees of the district nursing associations were formed by well-meaning but often very inexperienced individuals who could offer the time commitment involved. Most committees tried to enrol as many professional people as possible to help in the running of the district but, in many cases, those with the time and energy to fill the vital roles were not experts in the field.

The coordination of a network of independently managed district nursing associations required rules and structures. As early as 1893, a memorandum from Queen Victoria's Jubilee Institute for Nurses in London set out the relationship to be established between the superintendents and honorary secretaries of affiliated associations and the General Superintendent of the Queen's Institute. Much of this memorandum was about effective communication. It stressed the necessity to report all changes and decisions in writing with the correct format for correspondence.[15] In the days before modern infrastructures, the Queen's Institute was conscious of the need to keep the district nursing association committees up to date with developments in government policy. Annual visits from the inspector were followed by a letter to the honourable secretary, confirming how happy or otherwise the Queen's Institute was with progress and making any suggestions for improvements.

The inspectors tried to attend annual general meetings of district nursing associations or public meetings held for specific reasons. In towns near Dublin, the inspector, or even the superintendent, would endeavour to pop in to a sale of work or garden fete to show support. This was not often possible, however, given the great distances to cover and often a full calendar already.

In order for a district nursing association to be affiliated with the Queen's Institute, it had to show its financial prospects and demonstrate that it would be capable of providing permanent employment for the nurse.[16] Many district nursing associations were set up but failed due to lack of funds, lack of local interest or unspecified difficulties. The Queen's Institute was reluctant to send a nurse to a district if her tenure there was not secure. Districts were disaffiliated if there was any concern within the Queen's Institute that the nurse's salary would not be paid. The earliest example of an association that struggled from the start was Coole, Mayne and Kiltoom District Nursing Association in Westmeath. Set up in 1894, it was disaffiliated just three years later due to insufficient funds.

Disaffiliation from the Queen's Institute occurred when a district was no longer able to avail of a qualified nurse. This must have been quite a grim circumstance for committees, who had based much social kudos on their ability to sustain the service in their community. Occasionally a 'non-Queen's' nurse was employed by a district, and she was not always seen by the inspector as 'satisfactory'. This occurred more frequently during the period in 1909–1910 when so many districts were being set up by the Women's National Health Association (WNHA) groups that there was a resulting shortage of qualified nurses. Similar to the village nurse-midwives in England, some women without hospital experience were merely given a few months' training in St Laurence's Home before being allocated a district.[17] Called 'health workers', they were placed within communities with insufficient preparation and many of them quickly expressed their unhappiness with the work. Most districts which were supplied with a health worker were not successful and closed down within a two-to-four-year period. The exception to this was in the Lady Dudley island district of Arranmore in Donegal. Elizabeth Scully, a non-Queen's nurse, was appointed in 1916 and retired in 1945, after some sick leave, with a history of satisfactory reports.

Representatives from every district association attended the annual general meeting of the Queen's Institute in Dublin. The first meetings of the scheme were held in the hall of the College of Physicians, Kildare Street. Some representation came from very great distances, at a time when transport was not as comfortable as it is today. Travel and other expenses associated with these events did not seem to be a burden on the district nursing associations. Those attending stayed with friends and family when in Dublin for meetings. According to Maire Kennedy of Portmarnock District Nursing Association, it never occurred to anyone to claim personal expenses from their district nursing association for any costs incurred during these outings.[18]

Every year, annual reports – usually printed documents – and payment for continued affiliation with the Queen's Institute were required from each district nursing association.

Close relationships between secretaries of district nursing associations and the staff and council of the Queen's Institute developed over the years. There was, in the ordinary management of daily matters, much contact and regular visits by the Institute's inspectors to every district. Jean Cochrane, now living in Belfast but originally from Lifford in Donegal, remembers a lovely example of this relationship. Jean's grandmother set up the committee to raise funds for a Jubilee nurse for Lifford, Clonleigh and Castlefinn, County Donegal. It was, she says, initiated by the need for the dispensary doctor Dr Martin Coyne to have help in his huge district. Her grandmother, Mrs Boyd, then acted as the president of the committee. The secretary was Jean's mother. Together they set up the health club in 1932 and employed eight nurses before closing early in 1958. Jean Cochrane wrote to the authors to recall that Miss Kavanagh, the inspector for the Queen's Institute, always stayed in the Cochrane family home on visits to the district from Dublin and became great friends with Jean's mother. In return, the whole family would stay with Miss Kavanagh when they visited Dublin.[19]

In 1933 Miss Hart of Carrablagh, Portsalon Health Club, County Donegal was invited by the Countess of Kenmare, president of the Queen's Institute, to be a member of the institute's Executive Committee. There was a vacancy due to the death of Senator Lady

Desart. It was a great honour and must have been an enormous commitment for Miss Hart, as the committee met every month except during the summer and Christmas holidays. Even with the good train service from Dublin to Letterkenny at the time, it was a very long journey. Miss Hart had only just set up Fanad Health Club the year before. She was in the process, with Dr Ó Deagha, of setting up a county committee of Queen's nurses. Delving in the archives gives one the feeling that Miss Hart was probably good company, very efficient and a good addition to any working party. The large, and increasing, number of nurses in Donegal in the 1930s must also have influenced the institute to invite Miss Hart to join the committee as representative of that county.

RULES FOR A GOOD COMMITTEE

The fundamental principles for affiliation of a district nursing association and allocation of a permanent nurse were set out in a handbook for Queen's nurses, printed in 1924.

(a)   A uniform standard of qualification and training for the nurses employed;

(b)   Periodical inspection of nurses' work;

(c)   Carrying out of general sick nursing under the directions of the medical practitioners, and in accordance with the rules laid down;

(d)   Nursing of patients in their own homes who are unable to employ a private nurse, free nursing being given in case of necessity;

(e)   That the work shall be un-sectarian;

(f)   That the nurses shall not act as almsgivers.[20]

A Uniform Standard of Qualification and Training

The common standard of training and qualification was that dictated by the Queen's Institute.

Some of the very early district nursing associations and cottage hospitals had employed a non-Queen's nurse and were not affiliated until their nurse was replaced by one who was supplied by the Queen's Institute. In the normal course of events, once the district nursing association was established it immediately applied for a Jubilee nurse. This application would be assessed and the area inspected by an officer of the Queen's Institute and, if it was deemed appropriate, the association would receive its nurse.

Periodical Inspections

As mentioned above, every district was supervised by a visit from the superintendent or the inspector of the Queen's Institute at least once a year. Sometimes if a district was in difficulty, for whatever reason, extra visits were organised. In the early years of the scheme, the viceroy's wife, or other such dignitaries, would accompany the representative of the Queen's Institute on her perambulations around the country. The inspection provided valuable support to both the local committee and the nurse herself. It often took two days so that the Queen's Institute inspector could get a thorough understanding of the nurse's conditions and abilities. The inspector normally went on rounds with the nurse, gauging how popular, or otherwise, the nurse was with patients. The visit was regularly conducted around the time of the district nursing association's annual general meeting so that feedback could also be gained from the nurse's employers. It was customary for the inspector to stay with a member of the local committee during these visits as it saved the Executive Committee of the Queen's Institute many hotel bills.[21]

A lack of petrol during the 'Emergency' meant that the three motor cars which were usually used by the superintendents and inspectors in carrying out their visits had to be immobilised. Instead, they travelled by train and bus and were provided with a bicycle each, on which they had to cycle up to 30 or 40 miles a day, whatever the weather.[22] Back in head office, the report for each district was summarised in the Ledger of Jubilee Nurses Affiliated Branches usually with one or two words – 'satisfactory' or 'quite satisfactory' – unless further action was required by the Queen's Institute.

Directions of the Medical Practitioners

The dispensary doctor, medical officers and, in later years, general practitioners were a crucial element of 'outdoor' medical service in communities. Set up in 1851, the dispensary doctors were specifically provided to care for the poor and their service was administered on a ticket basis.[23] In 1920 there were 740 dispensary districts in Ireland and there was a trained midwife for every district in the country that year.[24]

In many districts, the arrival of the Queen's nurse was urged by the dispensary doctor. It is not surprising to find that doctors, and particularly their wives, were often active members of the district nursing association committees. Cork City Women's National Health Association was set up in 1907 by Dr Lucy Smith and Dr Olive Barry.

The connection between the local doctors, their family and the district nursing associations was logical because the Jubilee nurses' presence in the community would have assisted the doctor immeasurably. The Jubilee nurse was seen by the dispensary doctor as being of vital assistance to his work as there was often no pharmacy or clerical support. Mary Nolan, the widow of the last dispensary doctor for Mountcharles in County Donegal, said her husband could not have survived without the help of the Lady Dudley nurse. She said Dr Nolan had trained and then worked in a TB sanatorium before accepting what was then a secure job as dispensary doctor. The nurse and the dispensary were based in Frosses, an adjoining townland. As Frosses was subsidised from Dublin, there was no need for a local district nursing association committee. The doctor and his family were free of the obligation to maintain the nurse. Mrs Nolan's mother had been on the district nursing association committee for Enfield, County Meath, so she was aware of the constant need for fundraising. There was, according to Mary Nolan, always a cordial relationship between the nurses in Donegal and her husband and they held clinics in the dispensary two days a week, Mondays and Thursdays. As with the nurse, patients came to the doctor's house at all hours of the day and night.[25]

Dr Áine Sullivan in Cavan remembered a good working rapport between her father, the dispensary doctor, and the Jubilee nurse. In 1959, due to funding difficulties, disaffiliation of the district nursing association was suggested, and Áine remembers, even as a small child, the great distress that it caused in the household. The nurse would have been redirected to another district but her father, the already overworked doctor, would have been left without a greatly needed assistant.[26] Cavan had a public meeting and the district nursing association managed to limp along until 1967 through the fundraising efforts of the local community and the use of grants.

Free Nursing in Cases of Necessity

Many of the districts specified at the beginning of the affiliation process whether they were going to charge fees from patients who could afford them. It was up to the committee to fundraise in the manner with which they felt most comfortable. Some charged a small fee, as in Newtowncunningham, whose Jubilee nurse was known as the 'penny nurse'.[27] A frequent memory of nurses interviewed was of the patient, or a relative, sourcing a jar of funds from a hidden location, especially set aside for her visit. Midwifery charges were particularly important and patients felt it very essential to acknowledge their gratitude to the nurse with as large a payment as they could manage. All funds received by the nurse were given to the committee. It was recorded carefully as every penny was significant in the task of maintaining the service for the good of all. Sometimes there was a structure of successful fundraising which enabled a committee to instruct the nurse not to charge any fee. Towards the end of the Queen's Institute, when district nursing associations began to receive government grants, this was unnecessary as nurses then only accepted voluntary contributions. When the Queen's Institute ceased supplying nurses in 1968, many of the committees continued to provide voluntary services in their communities, looking after the elderly with meals, parties and outings. In 1963 at the Queen's Institute annual general meeting, delegates from all over the country were encouraged to do this in a lecture by Dr M.P. Flynn, County Medical Officer for Westmeath.[28]

Religion

The religion of the majority of the population, rather than that of the committee, was taken into consideration when sending a nurse to an area. While the perception was that the committees were Protestant and loyal to the English crown, this was far from the reality. There were many committees whose president was not a titled lady but was, in fact, the parish priest and most committees consisted of a happy mix of concerned people with no agenda other than the care of the poor in their community. Many committees organised to have pastors from several religions on the board. Most associations were acutely aware of the necessity for the nurse to treat all patients in a fair and equal manner based on need rather than money or religion.

The strictly non-sectarian nature of the Irish branch of the Queen's Institute came under pressure in the early stages of the organisation. In 1890, the Newry District Nursing Society for the Protestant Sick Poor in County Down presented a political dilemma for the Queen's Institute. Although this society did not deny care to sick Catholics, it can be assumed from the association's title that it favoured those patients of a Protestant persuasion. However, the situation was diplomatically managed by the superintendent, Miss Dunn, according to Mary Stokes in *A Hundred Years of District Nursing*.[29] The association was renamed the Newry District Nursing Society and it continued in its non-sectarian work. It was not officially affiliated until 1899. A house was purchased for the nurse in 1906. Nurse Rose McAlister was employed from 1910 to 1937 when she retired on a pension.

Nurses Shall Not Act as Almsgivers

In cases of desperate poverty, contrary to the English practice, Samaritan funds were established by district nursing associations whereby local individuals could donate towards the care of the underprivileged in the community. Most charity was dispensed in the form of extra milk, food or clothing supplied by members of the association rather than the nurse. In the case of tuberculosis patients, support for the family could be in the form of financial aid if the main wage earner was receiving treatment in a sanatorium. Upon inspection of Tralee District Nursing Association in 1928, Miss Colburn noted in her report that 'committee is turning nurse into almsgiver'. The situation was considered to be serious enough to warrant a second inspection just two months later. The inspector this time was Miss Kavanagh, who was satisfied that the committee members had taken over the responsibility of dispensing milk and clothing but also noted that the district's workload was extremely heavy and that a second nurse should be considered. No extra nurse was provided in the Tralee district and Nurse Hannah Roche remained there until her retirement in 1948.

THE COST OF A JUBILEE NURSE

The main expense for each district nursing association was the nurse's salary. This was decided by the committee, but a generous salary offering to the nurse influenced the Queen's Institute in their decision to affiliate an association. As the years passed it was recommended that an increase be given, particularly as the post of public health nurse was brought in and the working conditions of privately funded nurses would have to be kept to a similar standard as that set by the government-employed nurses. Recommendations were circulated to all district nursing associations and the nurse was often consulted to ensure that the association had followed through on this recommendation. Inspectors sometimes noted that the nurse had not been paid the new salary increase and this was seen as an indicator that a district nursing association was struggling financially.

An affiliation fee had to be paid annually to the Queen's Institute in order to allow the association to continue and a similar amount had to be contributed to the nurses' pension fund. Employers' share of the national health insurance, stamps or PRSI had to be paid and accident insurance was another annual expense to be administered. As the employers of the nurse, the secretary of the organisation, normally in collaboration with the treasurer, would have administrated all of this paperwork.

The Queen's Institute considered the provision of suitable accommodation for the nurse a very important duty for district nursing associations. Dr Seán Ó Deagha, the County Medical Officer, wrote to Miss Hart of Portsalon, County Donegal when she was setting up a district nursing association in the isolated area of Fanad. He warned that the Queen's Institute 'are very averse to permitting their nurses to reside in quarters which are neither comfortable nor healthy, though they do not always stick to the letter of the law in this matter, as, in certain areas, it is almost impossible to find decent accommodation'.[30] In April 1932 Miss Hart was again advised, this time by Miss Colburn of the Queen's Institute, not to pay too much for rooms without board, 'otherwise the total cost of the nurse exceeds our estimate'.[31] A cottage was provided for Nurse O'Dowd in Fanad. Nurse Clancy stayed in lodgings 'at a farm with very nice people, who are extremely good about my comings and goings at odd hours, and produce meals for me whenever I want them'.[32]

The availability of a furnished cottage, house or bungalow was often a deciding factor in the allocation of a nurse to a district. In several cases the president of the association provided this accommodation, initially at no cost, along with fuel for a fire and the attendance of a part-time maid. These were often part of the salary allocation for the nurse and, presumably, the comfort of the accommodation depended entirely on availability and the wealth and generosity of the district or its benefactors. The Queen's Institute fully supported district nursing associations that provided the cottage but even the provision of suitable accommodation did not guarantee that the arrangement would succeed in the long term. At Crumlin district in Antrim, the president of the committee, Mrs Pakenham, presented a 'beautiful home' to the association in 1906. The district had opened in 1901 but was disaffiliated by 1914. A much later district established in Carrickbyrne in Adamstown, Wexford only survived three years from 1947. This was in spite of the fact that one of the honourable secretaries on the committee had provided a cottage for the nurse.

If living conditions were not correct for the nurse, district nursing associations were frequently disaffiliated. The pressure this put on voluntary associations is mentioned frequently in reports and correspondence. Birr District Nursing Association, for instance, had great anxieties about the accommodation of their new nurse, Mary O'Hara. In the minutes of a meeting held on 13 September 1945, presided over and countersigned by Lady Rosse, the secretary wrote that the committee welcomed Miss O'Hara. Her salary and the half day she was due to take on Saturdays were discussed, as was the bill from the hotel where Nurse O'Hara was temporarily staying as the association was finding it very difficult to source comfortable permanent accommodation for her.

The Queen's Institute annual report for 1947 regretted that six district nursing associations were in abeyance and that 'in four of these it was impossible to secure lodgings, or a local house, as a residence for the nurse. In districts where cottages are not provided, there is no sense of security of tenure for the committee, as there is at present such demand for lodgings that landladies find a married couple cause less work than taking messages from patients for a nurse lodging in the house.'[33]

It was usually the duty of the secretary of each district nursing association to find and provide suitable accommodation for the nurses. It should be noted that in some areas the Jubilee nurse was closely associated with the village hospital and this relationship would have taken some of the stress from the district nursing association as the nurse's dual role would have easily justified her expense.

Another significant expense was transport which, for most nurses, was a pedal bicycle. In 1940 the Ballinasloe District Nursing Association had to pay for repairs to Nurse O'Grady's bicycle twice with a total spend of £16. 8/-. This was a very large expenditure considering the nurse's monthly salary was £12. 9/- 9d.[34] The *Queen's Nurses' Magazine* described the situation at the fishing village of Ardmore, County Waterford. The area was run by a district nursing association but was in such a poor region that establishment of the association was subsidised by the Queen's Institute.

> For some time after the nurse came she had no means of getting about except on foot, but she has now been provided with a bicycle. Already she has been sent for to distant cases in the hilly region round Ardmore where a short time ago no trained nurse had ever penetrated. Nurse Reidy can thus lay claim to being the first and pioneer nurse in this wild and very poor district.[35]

The lucky nurse in Enfield, County Meath was provided with a bicycle and a pony by her committee in 1907. At East Galway district, a bicycle, jennet and trap were made available for the nurse's use in the same year. Later committees purchased a car for the nurses and in some instances nurses brought their vehicle but were given an allowance to run it.

Committees of district nursing associations, usually those with origins in the Women's National Health Association, often had fiscal responsibility for mothers and baby clubs, a support system for new mothers and a place where nourishment could be provided and the health of babies and their siblings could be checked by the nurse. They would meet weekly at a community hall, which had to be rented or maintained. Talks on good nutrition and health matters were organised by the committee and often small gifts were given to the children at Christmas time. Dundrum District Nursing Association had a large prefabricated hall with a corrugated zinc roof which accommodated 300 people and was purchased by Lady Redmond in 1913 to hold classes, entertainments and clubs. Annie P. Smithson, the Jubilee nurse in Dundrum from 1917 to 1919, describes one of these baby clubs in the *Queen's Nurses' Magazine* of April 1918.

> Our Club is in a suburb of South Dublin. We have about 150 members and an average attendance of 80–100 mothers, 40 babies under one year old, and 60 under five. The Club meets every Monday at 3 p.m. The women pay one penny at the door and get a good tea; the babies are weighed, etc.; and short lectures are given to the mothers. There is a coal and boot club; we let them have Glaxo and Virol much below cost price (the Committee making up the deficiency); they can buy 'babies bundles' at 1s.8d and for 2s.6d we lend out maternity bags. Every second Monday our doctor attends, and on alternate Tuesdays we have a dental clinic for the school children between the ages of five and ten.[36]

After the nurse's salary, accommodation, heat and light had been accounted for, an important part of expenditure was the nurse's uniform. In most cases, the nurse was provided with her initial uniform and the important badge in the training home, and thereafter it was provided by the committee of her district. The Jubilee nurse had a very distinctive uniform and badge to differentiate her from the public authority health visitor or any other healthcare visitors in the community. Inspectors of districts sometimes noted that a nurse's uniform was untidy or worn, and this reflected badly on the entire organisation. Later, Jubilee nurses were given uniforms during training and the badge on assignment to a district.[37] The badge was returned on retirement or marriage of the nurse.

Longevity of District Nursing Associations

A strong committee often survived through many generations and the commitment was frequently passed from sister to sister or mother to daughter or daughters-in-law. Seventy-five district nursing associations lasted over 50 years. The district nursing associations to survive longest in Ireland were the association covering Dalkey, Killiney and Ballybrack, County Dublin and also Galway District Nursing Association, each surviving some 73 years. The district nursing association at Naas, County Kildare supported a Jubilee nurse for 72 years, while Dundalk, County Louth had a successful committee for 71 years. The Father Healy Association in Bray, County Wicklow; Powerscourt and Kilbride district, County Wicklow; Buncrana, County Donegal; Swords district, County Dublin; and Cahir district, County Tipperary all employed a Jubilee nurse for 70 years. The first Lady Dudley district in Ireland at Achill, County Mayo also lasted more than 70 years.

Many associations, however, lasted only a few years as often there was not the population or local support to provide sufficient financial sustenance for long-term employment of the nurse. Three associations survived just one year. In County Mayo, the Castlebar Women's National Health Association, formed in 1913, employed only one nurse before it folded. Ballinakill in 'Queen's County', now Offaly, founded a district nursing association and had a population of 500 but supported two nurses for less than one year. Finally, Silvermines District Nursing Association, County Tipperary closed due to 'lack of funds', with the nurse being transferred to Limerick. Fifty-eight associations did not survive for longer than ten years and many of these closed when their nurse had to leave because of marriage. Other associations were weak at the committee rank. Lauragh District Nursing Association, near Killarney, County Kerry, for example, opened in 1928 and closed four years later when the association's president, the dowager Marchioness of Lansdowne, died.

Districts were sometimes put into 'abeyance' whereby they were asked to reorganise themselves if possible. If the committee was able to improve finance, accommodation or overcome other obstacles upon this reorganisation, they were re-affiliated. Enniscorthy,

County Wexford opened in 1894 and closed in 1909 due to lack of funds. Money must have been found later in the year and they began again, this time remaining open for 52 years. The longest break between the reorganisation of associations within a town occurred in the Portarlington district. The district nursing association was affiliated under the leadership of secretaries Miss Cortellis and Miss Carr in 1914. They employed five nurses, two of whom left for military service in the First World War, and closed in 1921. Thirty-four years later, Portarlington received a Jubilee nurse. The new committee supervising this nurse survived from 1955 until 1966.

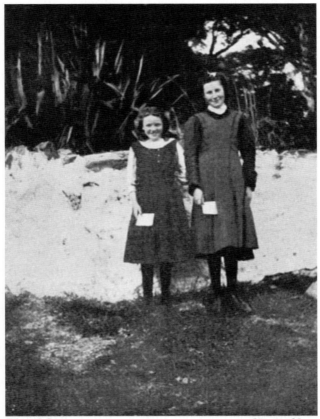

Photo by]   [*Lady Mayo*
Two Little Collectors in Co. Kerry
Two little collectors in Kerry, 1912. Door-to-door collecting was a vital part of fundraising for most district nursing associations.
Courtesy of the National Library of Ireland.

Branches of the Women's National Health Association moved, without any pause or disruption, into describing themselves as district nursing associations. However, others, such as Cashel, County Tipperary, still described themselves as a Women's National Health Association as late as 1950. Several associations also changed geographical boundaries, such as the Lady Dudley district of Recess, County Galway, which was founded in 1908 and amalgamated with Roundstone, Cashel district, which had begun in 1903. This new, larger district continued to operate until 1967. The Stillorgan, Newtown Park Avenue, Deansgrange and Kill o' the Grange District Nursing Association, founded in 1932 and covering a large area, was amalgamated with Foxrock in 1939. Foxrock and Stillorgan District Nursing Association had been founded in 1905 and employed thirteen nurses until it closed in 1966.

FUNDING

The difficulties involved in establishing, administering and funding nursing associations within communities is evident in the annual reports from all over the country. According to Florence Nightingale, 'the object of the association is to give first rate nursing to the poor sick at home (which they never have had) and this costs money'.[38] The sheer energy required to support the Jubilee nurse on her rounds was hard to appreciate. According to Miss Annie Michie, who was superintendent of the Queen's Institute in Ireland from 1912 to 1926:

> The work of the district nurses is little heard of, except in the few places where they are actually established. The chief reason is that there is not a large building to attract the public eye; no showy uniform, nothing but just quietly dressed women going amongst the poor in the various towns and country districts, trying to help those who in many instances are unable to help themselves.[39]

Several district nursing associations began with a bequest of money on the death of, or as a memorial to, a departed well-wisher, which enabled them to start up and often provided an income which helped with some of the running costs. The Carew bequest began in 1917 with £6,000 to provide a nurse for Kilcock, County Kildare.

In 1955 it was being administered by the Lady Dudley's Scheme but it benefited the three district nursing associations of Kilcock and Maynooth, County Kildare, and Trim, County Meath.[40]

According to the Queen's Institute report of 1947: 'The best nurse in the world cannot function adequately without the backing of her Committee, therefore we would pay tribute to the work done by committee Members and Collectors, remembering that the latter often have to pay a great number of visits to the homes of the people, before obtaining their annual contribution to the funds.'[41]

Fundraising was hard work but recording every penny and ensuring trust in the organisation was vital. Annual reports were usually very professionally presented and many were formal published documents with detailed accounts including donations of all sizes, from minuscule amounts to large contributions, and the results of fundraising events.[42] Explanations of the work done by the nurse in order to increase awareness and raise funds were printed occasionally. As mentioned above, the nurse was offered donations by grateful patients and did, in some districts, charge fees for her services, particularly from middle-class patients. The Queen's Institute felt that if people contributed small amounts to the committee regularly they were happy to avail of the service not as a charity.[43] Through the period studied, provident or 'stamp' schemes operated in some areas. The Donegal health clubs were based on the principle of regular contributions. The stamp schemes were a fashionable way of saving in the 1940s and the stamps were purchased from the Queen's Institute, or local district nursing association, for a penny each. One provident scheme had a slogan 'pay regularly when well, and be nursed free of charge when ill!' Most were voluntary and as a result not often successful because the nurse called to patients whether they had stamps or not.

Most financial support was collected door to door in the form of subscriptions from potential patients or from local businesses, by committee members. Small brown envelopes with the name of the district Jubilee Nurse Fund were handed out to residents and a parish, street or townland was allocated for each collector within their own district. This had the benefit of applying pressure to donate, particularly if the collector was known and liked. Collectors also knew from which homes it would be inadvisable to attempt to collect donations. Many former members of district nursing associations who were interviewed had mixed memories of the task of collecting money. In Enfield, County Meath, Mary Nolan (nee Prendergast) assisted her mother, a committee member of the local district nursing association, with door-to-door collections. As a young married woman, she would also be sent out to collect donations when she stayed with her parents on holidays. She remarked that women had almost hidden the money allocated for donation from themselves and had to climb up on chairs to reach the envelope on the tops of dressers. The people loved to see her coming and felt the 2/- a year was very well spent.[44] Fanad Health Club in Donegal was visited in 1935 by a journalist from the *Nursing Mirror and Midwives Journal*, who reported that 'many a farmer's wife saves the pennies by rigid economy in order to contribute a share for the family'.[45]

In rural areas where homes were isolated, people looked forward to the opportunity to call on neighbours and socialise. Door-to-door collections in some areas continued for many years after the Queen's Institute had closed, as some districts maintained the nurse. Reception of collectors varied greatly by district and period due to the sensitive nature of the activity – collecting money from one's neighbours had the potential to be a very awkward and uncomfortable experience or, conversely, a very rewarding one.

Much of the necessary finance was gathered during events such as whist drives (which were particularly popular), garden fêtes, carol singing, lectures, amateur theatre evenings, raffles, tea parties, bake and plant sales, or other sales of work including the important jumble sales. Flag days (usually held in the main street of large towns over two days) involved selling a little paper flag on a pin for a donation to the cause. The Queen's Institute inspector in 1957 reported that the district nursing association at Annamoe, County Wicklow, formed in 1933, had no funds to pay the nurse and was going to hold a fête because 'the committee were anxious to continue'. Annamoe District Nursing Association closed in 1958.

An open garden day would seem a relatively effortless fundraiser once the garden was attractive. A large envelope of correspondence and paper cuttings were donated to the Donegal Archives in Lifford. They describe a short period around the time of the setting

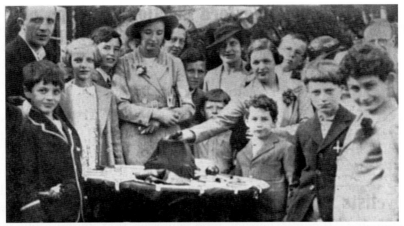

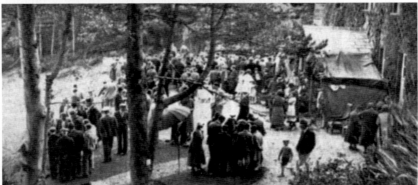

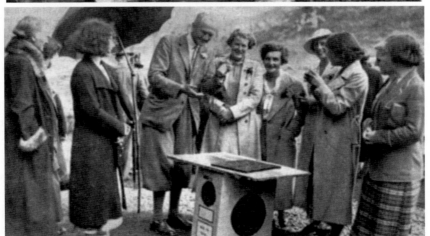

The weather was kind in Carrablagh in 1936 when Miss Hart held a most successful garden fête to support the two new jubilee nurses in the district of the Fanad Peninsula. Courtesy of Copyright Donegal County Archives, P/27.

up of Fanad Health Club in 1931. The correspondence includes items not normally kept, such as permits from the Garda Síochána to hold flag days. Handmade and printed posters for fairs, carnivals, céilís and jumble sales also feature. This file also contains a letter from the Londonderry Lough Swilly Railway Company, which was putting on a special bus service for an open garden day at Carrablagh Garden and had handbills printed to advertise the event. If the weather turned out to be inclement the company would, of course, not offer the service. As it turned out the day was windy, but dry; buses came from Derry and Letterkenny but the motor boat from Buncrana could not run. It was a very successful fundraising day as 200 people attended and 'tea was daintily served by a willing band of helpers in the verandah'.[46] Carrablagh Garden has a wonderful sheltered microclimate, overlooking a small picturesque cove, and is at present being lovingly restored to its original splendour.[47] In 1935 Miss Hart opened her gardens for another day. The result was £6. 11/- from the gate, £5. 12/- at tea and £5 odd at the side show. This was a very respectable outcome from the 121 people who attended on a very fine day. A golf competition raised £6 that year and the flag day in Portsalon Links on 4 August was £2. 18/- 5d. The photographs from the Garden fête held in Carrablagh depict a lovely, enjoyable day. The records for Miss Hart seem to end at that stage.[48]

The nurses' dance in Newtowncunningham, County Donegal, held in November or early December, was the highlight of the year. Ladies made their dresses months in advance and it was all anyone discussed for weeks. Ballinasloe, County Galway likewise loved their nurses' dance and in Cavan, formal dress was required for a very popular evening.[49] The nurses' dance or ball was an opportunity for one to be seen, and even photographed, in style with hair properly set and fingernails polished.

A consistent bureaucratic element which impacted on the work of both the nurse and the committee were the reports which had to be regularly presented to the Queen's Institute and the local community. Some rural districts were entitled to receive funding from organisations like the Benevolent Society of St Patrick (known as the Irish Peasantry Society), based in Charing Cross Road, London. The grant was not large but required a lot of paperwork and many rules had to be adhered to before it was approved each year. Another grant was available to some of these district nursing associations from the Irish Lights Office, D'Olier Street, Dublin.[50]

For many districts, the possibility of raising funds from 'public monies' under the Child Welfare Act, school nursing programmes and tuberculosis schemes existed. The granting of such funds depended on the efficiency of the secretary of each associa-tion in finding out about and applying for the available grants. Sligo District Nursing Association (1896–1960), under secretary Kathleen Ardill, made consistent petitions during its existence to obtain funds through grants for the child welfare and mater-nity scheme. Sending annual reports and grant applications, many handwritten, from the late 1920s to the late 1930s, Kathleen Ardill added in the comment section of a form that 'this is the only mater-nity or child welfare carried out in Sligo – the work is very much appreciated by the mothers who carry out the nurse's advice'. In 1929 the nurse visited 3,120 cases in her work during the year.[51] Mrs Kilduff, honorary secretary of Ballinasloe District Nursing Association, County Galway, also wrote regularly to the Custom House, Local Government Department in Dublin, in long hand, often apologising for the delay in sending the annual reports. The annual accounts, also handwritten, included all grants received on the basis of tuberculosis schemes and from the School and Local Government Department grants in1940. The total grants came to £73 while total income for that year was £204, raised through subscriptions, donations and the dance.[52]

Not all district nursing association secretaries were as success-ful, or prepared to commit the necessary time and energy to the bureaucracy, at securing grants from local health offices or the Department of Local Government in the Custom House in Dublin. In 1950, of the remaining 194 associations, 188 were receiv-ing subsidies from state or local authorities. These figures do not include the Lady Dudley's Scheme.[53]

In 1968, the Queen's Institute ceased all training and disburse-ment of Jubilee nurses. Some district nursing associations chose to continue in operation following the cessation of activity by the Queen's Institute in order to continue the employment of the local Jubilee nurse. Several continued until 1974.

Sources

Much of the information in this chapter is derived from the register of all district nursing associations whose jubilee nurse was affiliated with the Queen's Institute. The *Jubilee Nurses, Affiliated Branches* were recorded in three journals in longhand. These records are now in the safekeeping of Bord Altranais at UCD Archives, Dublin. Access is limited due to the personal nature of the registers.

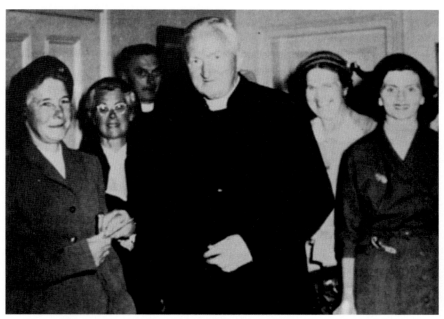

Nurse Jane Kelly of Galway receiving a presentation from Bishop Michael Browne and members of the Committee of St. Joseph's Nursing Society, 1954. Courtesy of Kenny's Bookshop, County Galway.

Notes

1   Jubilee Nurses, Affiliated Branches, P220/28–30, vols 1, 2, 3. An Bord Altranais Archives, UCD.

2   QVJIN, Annual Report, 1929, p. 9. National Archives, Dublin

3   Correspondence between Miss Hart, Portsalon, Co. Donegal and Dr Ó Deagha, Coiste Sláinte Dhún na nGall, 12 October 1931, Box P27/10. Donegal Archives, Lifford, Co. Donegal.

4   QVJIN, Annual Report, 1947. National Archives, Dublin.

5   Miss F.H Aylward, 'Domiciliary Nursing and Public Health Work', *Irish Nursing News* (December/January 1955), p. 4. This was part of the

transcript of a speech given to a world congress of nursing in Quebec, Canada in 1954.

6   QVJIN, Annual Report, 1935, National Archives, Dublin.

7   *Queen's Nurses' Magazine* (May 1906), p. 19, The Queen's Nursing Institute, London.

8   *Sligo Champion*, 1936. From Department of Health files M26/12. National Archives, Dublin.

9   Lady Dudley's Scheme, Annual Report, 1911, National Library, Dublin.

10   The UNRRA was set up before the United Nations by 44 countries, led by the United States of America, to provide shelter and relief to refugees all over Europe between 1943 and 1947. It was most active in 1945.

11   Dr Coey-Bigger, Address to the General Nursing Council, 13 February 1920, *The Journal of the Statistical and Social Inquiry Society*, p. 50. National Library, Dublin.

12   Interview with Bernie Hartery, Phyllis Fennelly and Anne Connolly in Waterford, Friday 12 November 2010.

13   Sir Edward Coey Bigger, MD, 'Public Health and Medical Services', in William G. Fitzgerald (ed.), *The Voice of Ireland* (Dublin: John Heywood Ltd, 1924), pp. 355–61.

14   QIDN, Annual Report, 1935, p. 20. National Archives, Dublin.

15   'Memorandum for Superintendents and Honorary Secretaries of Affiliated Associations in Dublin and throughout Ireland, regarding their relationship towards the general Superintendent of the Institute in Ireland' (1893). The Queen's Nursing Institute, London.

16   Pamphlet published for Queen Victoria's Institute for Nurses 1913. The Queen's Nursing Institute Archives, Wellcome Library, London.

17   Carrie Howse, 'The Development of District Nursing in England, 1880–1925', *Nursing History Review*, vol. 15, pp. 65–94.

18   Mrs M. Kennedy, Portmarnock DNA, Co. Dublin. Telephone interview, 30 January 2012.

19   Letter to the authors from Jean Cochrane, Belfast, 30 May 2011.

20   *Handbook for Queen's Nurses, by Some Queen's Superintendents* (London: Scientific Press Ltd, 1924), pp. 12–13. The Queen's Nursing Institute, London.

21   Ibid.

22   QIDN, Annual Report, 1941, p. 6.

23   Ruth Barrington, *Health Medicine and Politics in Ireland 1900–1970* (Dublin: Institute of Public Administration, 1987).

24   Bigger, 'Public Health and Medical Services'.

25   Interview with Mrs Mary Nolan, Mountcharles, Co. Donegal, 12 August 2011.

26   Interview with Dr Á. Sullivan, Cavan, 6 September 2011.

27   Group interview in the home of Mr and Mrs Chance, Manorcunningham, Co. Donegal, 11 August 2011.

28   *Irish Times*, 14 March 1963, p. 6. Report on the AGM of the Queen's Institute in the Overend Hall, Leeson Street, Dublin. Irish Times Archives.

29   Mary Stocks, *A Hundred Years of District Nursing* (London: Allen & Unwin, 1960).

30   Correspondence between Miss Hart, Portsalon, Co. Donegal and Dr Ó Deagha, Coiste Sláinte Dhún na nGall, 2 February 1932, Box P27/10. Donegal Archives, Lifford, Co. Donegal.

31   Correspondence between Miss Hart, Portsalon, Co. Donegal and QIDNI Dublin, Box P27/10. Donegal Archives, Lifford, Co. Donegal.

32   'In Wildest Donegal', *The Nursing Mirror and Midwives Journal* (12 October 1935), p. 28.

33   QIDN, Annual Report, 1947, p. 6. National Archives, Dublin.

34   Correspondence and annual reports from Mrs K. Kilduff, Ballinasloe, Co. Galway. Department of Health files, M104/8. National Archives, Dublin.

35   *Queen's Nurses' Magazine* (May 1904), p. 18. The Queen's Nursing Institute, London.

36   *Queen's Nurses' Magazine* (May 1918), pp. 43–4.

37   Interview with Bernie Hartery, Phyllis Fennelly and Anne Connolly in Waterford, Friday 12 November 2010.

38   Florence Nightingale, 'Introduction' in William Rathbone, *The History and Progress of District Nursing* (London: Macmillan, 1890).

39   Lady Russell and Miss Michie, 'Address to the General Nursing Council', *The Journal of the Statistical and Social Inquiry Society*, 13 February 1920, p. 53. National Library, Dublin.

40   Lady Dudley's Scheme, Annual Report, 1955, p. 12. Donegal Archives, Lifford, Co. Donegal.

41   QIDN, Annual Report, 1947, p. 7. National Archives, Dublin.

42   Many of these reports are in the Department of Health files, National Archives, Dublin.

43   QIDN, Annual Report, 1929. National Archives, Dublin.

44   Interview with Mrs Nolan, Mountcharles, Co. Donegal, 12 August 2011.

45   'In Wildest Donegal', p. 28.

46   Unidentified newspaper cuttings, 16 September 1932, Miss Hart, Portsalon, Co. Donegal. Box P27/10, Donegal Archives, Lifford, Co. Donegal.

47   Carrablagh House and Gardens are Number 17 on the Garden Trail of Donegal. Visiting is limited.

48   Correspondence, scrapbook and newspaper cuttings, Miss Hart, Portsalon, Co. Donegal. Box P27/10, Donegal Archives, Lifford, Co. Donegal.

49   Interview with Dr Á. Sullivan, Cavan on 6 September 2011.

50   Correspondence, 7 July 1932, Miss Hart, Portsalon, Co. Donegal. Box P27/10, Donegal Archives, Lifford, Co. Donegal.

51   Department of Health files, M26/12. National Archives, Dublin.

52   Ibid., M104/8.

53   Ibid., M100/150.

CHAPTER 4

Profiles of District Nursing Associations and Queen's Nurses

DISTRICT NURSING ASSOCIATIONS

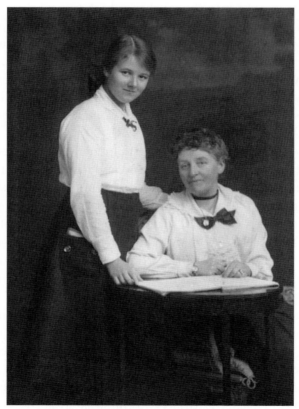

Lily and Naomi Overend. Both Lily and her daughter Naomi were invited to participate on the committee of the district nursing association in Dundrum. Fundraising was an activity in which the whole family participated, as was the case for many others in the area. Courtesy of the Airfield Trust, Dundrum.

Dundrum District Nursing Association

In February 2005 a brown box labelled 'Jubilee Nurse' was discovered by the author in the small archive room of Airfield House,
Dundrum, Dublin 14. The box contained a very large collection
of annual reports for a district nursing association that lasted
from 1898 to the very end of the scheme in 1968. It also held two
substantial leather-bound ledgers – one red, with gold lettering,
titled 'WNHA St Joseph's Baby Club Dundrum' and the other
black, with gold lettering, titled 'Dundrum, Sandyford & Milltown
Branch of WNHA'. The box also included random correspondence
from the Queen's Institute and a number of small printed card
receipts for money collections. Reading the contents of this small
box gives an insight into the workings of a typical district nursing
association over more than half a century. The people who gathered these reports and letters were involved as active participants,
in several roles, in the work of the district nursing association
for many years. It reflects the involvement and interest in their
community of two generations of women and their dedication and
willingness to work hard to ensure proper care for the sick and
young of the parish.

The Overend family lived permanently at Airfield House,
Dundrum from 1905. Trevor Overend and his wife Lily (nee Butler)
had two daughters – Letitia (1880–1974) and Naomi (1900–1993),
who remained in the house until their deaths. The two sisters left
the house, gardens and small farm in trust for the education of the
people of Dundrum. Women of their class were expected to be
socially involved in good works from early childhood. As children,
they organised parties to fundraise and gave some of their pocket
money to the 'children's league of pity', the children's branch of
the National Society for the Prevention of Cruelty to Children. As a
young woman in the early 1920s, and with the help of her friend Dr
Ella Webb, Letitia Overend played a vital role in the setting up and
maintenance of the Sunshine Home in Foxrock which prevented
many thousands of children from being permanently deformed by
the disease of rickets. Letitia Overend was so active in St John's
Ambulance that in 1955 she was awarded their highest honour as
Dame Justice of the Order of St John.

During both world wars, and particularly the Great War of 1914 to 1918, the family were very active in their support for the soldiers suffering on the front. They gathered hand-knit socks, bandages, cigarettes and other home comforts from the community, which were then sent to the rat-infested trenches through the Dundrum branch of the War Hospital Supply Depot. The head office of the War Hospital Supply Depot was based at 14 Merrion Square, Dublin and Letitia worked as a member of staff, packing and sending bales of hospital supplies all over Europe. She continued to work in a voluntary management capacity in this organisation for many years. As well as many unmarked personal acts of charity and kindness, the Overend sisters were involved with the Dublin Society for the Prevention of Cruelty to Animals, the Alexandra Guild and, lastly, the Dundrum/Ballinteer District Nursing Association.

The first committee for a district nursing association in the area was set up as the Milltown, Windy Arbour, Clonskeagh and Dundrum District Nursing Association in 1889. With a population of 1,158 the area needed one nurse. They were affiliated to the Queen's Institute in 1899. The honorary secretaries were Mrs T. Edmondson and Miss V. Henshaw. The association was given a grant of £20, did not charge fees or offer a midwifery service. They did not provide a cottage or house to the nurse but, similar to many of the early associations, only provided board, lodgings and laundry. Their first nurse, Elizabeth Naughton, had qualified at St Patrick's Home and came straight to the district in 1899. She was joined by Kathleen Browne from Limerick in 1900. Both nurses, who received 'satisfactory' reports, appear to have been with the association until its disaffiliation in 1909. This first association closed without explanation but in most instances where an association closed early it was because of committee or financial problems.[2] Later, Mrs Henshaw appears in the second annual report of the Dundrum, Sandyford and Milltown branch of the Women's National Health Association. She was, like the Overend sisters, a very dedicated collector of subscriptions until the 1950s when she was elected president of the association. Miss Henshaw died in 1960. It was noted in the foreword of the annual report that year that

… it had been some time since she was well enough to share in the business of the committee but for many years she, with her sisters Mrs Pringle and Mrs Orpen, were the mainstay of the association. Her death breaks a link with the early days. It is good to know the hard work of those years still bears fruit.[3]

This pattern of mothers, sisters and other family members together involved in raising funds and supporting the Jubilee nurse is repeated in many of the districts analysed.

The Queen's Institute's list of affiliated branches includes the second nursing association for the area encompassing Dundrum, Sandyford, Milltown and Clonskeagh, County Dublin. It was a branch of the Women's National Health Association. Lady Aberdeen was still in residence in Dublin Castle, and association with her projects was deemed a very acceptable pursuit for ladies. The branch was set up in 1912 but was only affiliated with the Queen's Institute in 1914 when it employed a qualified Queen's nurse. The population was 5,000 and the first secretary was Miss Ingham, shortly replaced by Mrs King. The association agreed to pay the nurse £90 inclusive salary in 1914. In 1916, the salary was £74 excluding fire, light and lodging, which was free, and by March 1926 the nurse's inclusive salary was £170.[4] Mrs R.V. Pringle, who succeeded Mrs King, continued as secretary until 1949 and died very shortly after she retired from the position. Mrs Hudson Kinhan took the post for a relatively short while, as did Mrs Ganly. The final secretary was Mrs J.M. Eyre, who continued until the association closed in 1968. Lady Redmond, the first president of the association, was very actively involved until her death in 1941, at which point Mrs Lily Overend took over as president. The position of president seems to have become symbolic rather than a working role by that stage. The first page of the annual reports usually detailed the committee members. They show movement within the committee over the years. Roles of treasurer, secretary or vice-president changed but the names remained fairly consistent. This would indicate that they were fortunate with longstanding nurses who did not need much management by the committee.[5]

The Overends' first involvement with the district nursing service is vague. Scrutiny of the two large handwritten ledgers found at Airfield House show that the Women's National Health Association ledger began in 1912 and the St Joseph's Baby Club ledger began recording in 1914 and ended in 1946. Except for occasional entries, both books seem to have been accounts of the Dundrum branches of the Women's National Health Association and Baby Club only, recorded usually in the hand of Letitia Overend. Letitia never became a member of the committee, unlike her mother Lily and sister Naomi. Letitia has described lists, on two pages, in the WNHA ledger of income and expenditure for 19 March 1913 as 'Analysis for Meeting'. The lists of income and expenditure for the area correspond to those printed on the annual general report.[6] One can presume from this that each parish had people who were not necessarily on the committee but were assigned to assist the treasurer for the whole district with collections of subscriptions, donations, all expenses and accurate recordkeeping. The administration of the association was taken seriously and not one penny donated went missing or was spent without due consideration.

In the Airfield archive the first published record of the new district nursing association is the second report of the branch and it is for the year ending 1914. It was called the *Women's National Health Association, Dundrum, Milltown and Sandyford Branch.* The president was Lady Redmond, Gortmore, Dundrum. The three vice-presidents were Mrs Gibbon, Taney Rectory, Dundrum, Mrs O'Brien and Mrs Barrington. Miss Cotton, Dromartin Hill, as honorary treasurer has been added by hand to the inside cover in Lily's handwriting. Miss Cotton was a good friend of Letitia Overend as she mentions many visits for social and personal gatherings at Miss Cotton's in her daily diary. The Overend family contributed £1 in the year 1914. While documentation continued in the handwritten ledgers, several printed annual reports are missing and only began to be regularly collected from 1921.[7]

Both ladies were ordinary members of the association until 1925 when Lily became a member of the committee of the, now named, Milltown, Dundrum branch. A list of 54 subscriptions collected by Mrs Lily Overend is included in the printed annual report that year. Every subscriber is named and the amount donated is listed. Mrs Overend's total amount collected came to £34.13/- 0d. These lists appear almost competitive. In the same year Mrs R.W. Pringle, who was honorary secretary, collected £8. 3/- 0d. and her sister

Miss Henshaw collected £7. 5/- 0d. Mrs Musters, also a committee member, collected £4. 4/- 0d. Miss Yeats, a former committee member, collected a mere £3. 17/- 6d. Two more committee members, Mrs Randal and Mrs Meehan, collected £3 and £1. 8/- 0d. respectively. Finally, Miss Vera McCaughey, an ordinary member, collected 15/- 6d. Subscribers at this time tended to be neighbours, friends and family of the committee. It can be seen that for many years the Overends were a dominant force in raising funding through subscriptions. As the years progressed it became harder to collect subscriptions and the committee began to rely on business people, professionals such as the local doctor and solicitor, banks and manufacturing companies in the area. As valued customers it may have been hard to refuse the committee members' requests to support the community nurse. Mrs Lily Overend was made president in 1941 on the death of Lady Redmond and continued until her death in 1945. Naomi was elevated to the committee and she became president on the death of Miss Henshaw in 1960; she was the last president of the association.[8] A common factor in many district nursing associations was that individuals rarely retired and usually stayed on, in some capacity, until they died. The voluntary assistance of people was valued irrespective of age.

Despite constant fundraising efforts, the committee ran into trouble in 1942 when the inspector of the Queen's Institute reported the 'financial position unsatisfactory'. Miss Aylward, the superintendent, attended the annual meeting of the district nursing association in November that year, as was quite common when there were concerns. Nurse Jones was also retiring at this time. She noted that 54 people attended the meeting. By 1956, Inspector Delaney was able to report that the funds were fairly good and the committee was getting new council houses for the nurses.[9]

Published annual reports of the Milltown, Dundrum District Nursing Association are an interesting study in themselves. These reports were several pages long, stapled with a cover and professionally printed on good quality paper. They document, in addition, the changing fashions of typescript, descriptive detail and social mores from 1914 to 1967. They show from year to year the changing committee due to illness and death and the difficulties, and successes, in fundraising. Some years there were multiple copies, possibly because one of the Overends had organised the printing of the report itself. Every year the report enumerated the work of the nurses and reflected the social and economic difficulties of patients from before the foundation of the state through to the evolution of the health boards. By the early 1950s the name of the association had changed from Women's National Health Association Milltown and Dundrum Branch to Dundrum and Ballinteer District Nursing Association. In 1960 it was called the Dundrum District Nursing Association but had responsibility for the areas of Ballinteer, Churchtown, Beaumont, Windy Arbour, Goatstown, Roebuck, Mount Merrion and Clonskeagh. It was just as well there were two nurses at that time. These reports were distributed to all members, the health authorities and county council. They show the accounts, outlining donations, fundraising successes and all the expenses in minute detail. It is a catalogue of the generosity and public spirit of the people of the district.

An example of the care, expense and attention to detail which was employed in preparing the annual report is demonstrated in the ninth report for the year ending March 1921. It was professionally printed with a grey soft-back cover on high-quality paper. It began with a page that lists the president, Lady Redmond, and vice-presidents. The 23 members of the committee are named and their addresses included. The president's report is over two pages in length and her contribution can be synopsised as a big thank you to everyone involved. Emphasis is placed on preventative work with extra nutrition and clothes administered to mothers and babies through the baby club. Nurse Healy is welcomed and appreciated. Finally, the Ladies Association of Charity, Dundrum are thanked most sincerely. The next section is a list of six 'Contributors of Clothing'; Mrs Switzer and Miss Yeats – both of notable families – are among this number. 'Nurse Healy's Report' is interesting due to the vast amount of work she carried out that year, including 4,423 general visits, 822 tubercular visits and 3,406 child welfare visits. The nurse notes, among many different elements of her work, the deaths of an infant (under one year) and one child (under two years). The section headed 'Samaritan Work' lists the donators of such things as food, milk, virol, Oxo, eggs and old linen (a lot of old linen) a mackintosh and nursing appliances (bed pans, feeding cups and air pillow, etc.). The 'Dental Clinic' report outlines that the clinic was held twice monthly for the benefit of the children attending the national schools of Dundrum and Milltown districts. The nurse assisted the dentist to examine 432 children (boys and girls) and 156 cases had to be treated at the clinic. Half of the expenditure for this department was refunded by the National Board. The 'Honorary Treasurers Report' notes an increase that year of baby club members from 154 to 170. They received a government grant of £68. 13/- 11d.[10]

Correspondence recovered from the Airfield archives included letters from the Queen's Institute congratulating the Overends on successful fundraising events, particularly their garden fêtes. An effusive letter of 1 June 1934 from the superintendent, Miss Colburn, congratulated everyone, apologised for being unable to attend, and she 'hoped you all agree that the magnificent result achieved made up for the time, thought and labour'. Not all garden parties were blessed with such clement weather, however, and in 1956 they had a splendid result of £14. 8/- 6 considering the poor conditions. The superintendent for Ireland wrote saying how much she enjoyed the day and seeing their beautiful cows.[11] The Overend sisters were quite famous for their herd of jersey cows, whose creamy milk they sold in the neighbourhood. The Overends, and the committee, were acutely aware of the need for such funds as Nurse Jones retired after 25 years' service in 1950. Like many of her colleagues she had remained single to carry on the work. As a voluntary committee they would never have been in a position to guarantee the payment of a pension continuously, to any nurse, even one as loved as Nurse Jones.

The first nurse in the Dundrum, Sandyford, Milltown and Clonskeagh Women's National Health Association branch was Nurse Gumbrielle, who had to leave after one year due to ill health. She was replaced by the qualified Jubilee nurse Lily Lyndon. Nurse Lyndon was from Cork city and had trained in the Mater and St Laurence's Home for training district nurses, becoming a Queen's nurse in 1913. Her first appointment was as a temporary nurse for Dundrum in December 1913, which became permanent in February 1914. She asked for leave of absence after the war in 1917. The Queen's Institute reports said she was 'much liked by her committee and patients'. After a year she re-joined the institute and was sent to Cork where she stayed until 1920.[12]

Nurse Lyndon was replaced by Annie P. Smithson, who had been stationed at Ballina, County Mayo. She asked for a transfer because she believed she may be in danger as she was on a list of 'Sinn Féin' supporters in the RIC barracks just after the 1916 Rising. Nurse Annie Smithson's career is considered in detail in Chapter 1. In her autobiography, she describes her time in Milltown, Dundrum as a happy one back in her native Dublin. It was 'a large scattered district with much cycling, but to me after my years in the country, it was child's play'.[13] In the *Queen's Nurses' Magazine*, Annie P. describes her work and the organisation of a Christmas party for the Baby Club. She praises the generosity of the committee in providing food supplements and clothing parcels to distribute to the members of the baby club, who met every Monday at 3 p.m. For the party, the members of the committee helped with making the tea, providing a decent meal for the 'kiddies' and a present for every child.[14] Annie, and many Jubilee nurses in the country, were shocked by the influenza epidemic of 1918, and in Milltown, Dundrum it was remembered vividly. She describes having four in a bed and the next day one may be dead. On duty night and day, she succumbed to the disease herself and there was no nurse to replace her. She stayed until 1919 and left because of conflict with the committee, who were traditionally loyal to the crown of England or, as Annie described them, 'a strongly loyalist committee'. Annie had become more and more nationalist in her views and was so 'full of enthusiasm that I did not seem to mind what might happen to me in consequence'.[15] Her first novel *Her Irish Heritage*, published in 1918 – though not read by the ladies, according to Annie – was perceived as rather nationalist and led to tensions. It was the hanging of the Sinn Féin flag out the window of the nurse's cottage that shocked her committee. As mentioned previously, the nurse's relationship with the committee was pivotal for mutual support. That nurse Smithson disagreed politically with the committee in a time of such conflict was enough; displaying her affiliations openly was unforgivable, leading to insurmountable tensions. She was replaced by a nurse who had returned from the war in Europe and, according to Annie, was popular with the committee because she had lovely stories of 'nursing British Tommies'.[16] Nurse Ellen Healy went to school in Killarney, County Kerry. She trained as a nurse and midwife in Belfast and completed her training as a Jubilee nurse in St Laurence's Home in Parnell Square, Dublin in 1914. She began her career in Westport, County Mayo and as a temporary nurse in Stamullen, County Meath until she went for military service. She must have been exceptionally well liked by the committee because on leaving Dundrum in 1925 for 'other work', Mrs Pringle, the secretary, put a note in her records with the Queen's Institute: 'Nurse Healy's work has been carried out in a most efficient way. Her influence on the mothers has been splendid. We part with her with regret and wish her every success in her new sphere.'[17] This uncommon note by a district nursing association committee member in the records of the Queen's Institute shows an exceptional rapport between the Dundrum committee and the Queen's Institute.

Nurse Margaret Jones was from County Monaghan and trained as a general nurse in Belfast. She graduated as a Queen's nurse from St Laurence's Home in 1909. She was described on leaving her training as 'reliable, considerate and has plenty of common sense'.[18] Milltown, Dundrum District Nursing Association was her second post following a period in the district of Midleton, County Cork. Nurse Jones took over from Nurse Healy in 1925 and stayed in Dundrum until she retired in 1950 with a pension from the Queen's Institute. Annual inspections of the district by the Queen's Institute were almost completely satisfactory throughout the 25 years of Nurse Jones's time. Occasionally the institute sent a representative to the annual general meeting at the time of inspection and in 1943 Inspector Aylward noted the committee was not paying the new scale of salary.[19] Fundraising must have been difficult in periods of stress such as the 'emergency in Europe', which led to deep poverty, especially in urban parts of Ireland. Annual reports from the committee were always satisfied with Nurse Jones's work.

In 1949 the question of a second nurse was raised with the County Medical Officer. There were concerns that it was unsuitable that the Jubilee nurse attended both midwifery cases and infectious cases. There was a midwife in the area employed by the Rathdown Board of Assistance. In 1953 a letter to the county council medical officer noted how much the nurse's work had increased due to the number of houses recently built in the area. A new Cyclemaster bicycle was provided and a grant of £50 towards the baby clinic. A letter from the secretary of the Department of Health sent to the Dublin County Medical Officer set out the services being provided for the area in November 1956. The letter stated that the District Nursing Association was employing one nurse at that time. It was prepared to raise the £900–£1,000 needed for a second nurse if a grant of £740 was provided for a temporary period, possibly one year. In 1957 it was agreed that two dispensary nurses would have meant a large increase in local authority expenditure.[20] The decision to supplement the District Nursing Association to let them provide another Jubilee nurse was pragmatic.

After Nurse Jones retired, Nurse Kathleen McConigly arrived, with her own car, and was given an extra £1 per week to enable her to cover more ground.[21] She stayed for one year before being transferred to County Donegal where she stayed until 1953. Nurse Catherine Foskin, originally from Mullingar, stayed a year and resigned for marriage. She was followed by Nurse Maura McLoughlin who was from Dundalk in County Louth. Nurse McLoughlin is one of the nurses featured in Chapter 1. Arriving in 1952, Dundrum was her first district and she stayed until 1957 when she resigned to get married. Mrs Kilmartin, nee McLoughlin, was still nursing in Dundrum in 1967 when the Jubilee nursing service was discontinued. After the service was disbanded, worries of the committee, described in letters to the Department of Health, were, for the most part, concerned with Nurse Kilmartin and Nurse Theresa Killalea's entitlements to continued employment or retirement funding. Nurse Killalea had begun in the district in 1958. She was a Galway woman trained in England and at the National Maternity Hospital Dublin. She qualified from St Patrick's Home in 1952 and had been transferred from four districts in a short period of time. By the time she reached Dundrum the superintendent noted that 'she had been rather unsettled and was [now] more contented'.[22] Dundrum by 1957 had two nurses for the district. These were Nurse Killalea and a series of temporary nurses during Nurse Kilmartin's two-year leave of absence. Nurse Killalea was offered a public health post in 1968.[23] As was the norm with the Queen's Institute official records, there is no mention of Nurse McLoughlin after her marriage. Maura Kilmartin, nee McLoughlin, contacted us with her memories of Jubilee nursing in Dundrum and her period as a public health nurse in the same district. Mrs Kilmartin's daughter Catherine still serves the community of Dundrum/Ballinteer as a district nurse and so the continuity of care endures.[24]

The generosity of the district nursing association committee cannot be exaggerated, especially in the early part of the century when Ireland had very little social support, desperate poverty and rampant tuberculosis. Lady Redmond was most unstinting, with large individual donations and purchases such as the wooden structure that housed the baby club, initially in Dundrum, and subsequently moved to Milltown. It was eventually considered dangerous and sold in 1941 by the committee the year after Lady Redmond died. The Carnegie Library offered temporary accommodation at the time. The Samaritan funds mentioned above were a monthly demand on resources and energy. The most obvious largesse was of time. Someone had to compose and organise the printing and distribution of the many leaflets and flyers for the association. Leaflets in the collection provided explanations of the nurse's activities and service to the community. This was essential in order to make the public aware and to garner support throughout the entire period of the association. Door-to-door collections were usually conducted in autumn and winter by the committee members and recorded in the annual accounts. The nurse did not charge for her services but a donation was often expected from those who could afford it. Many more leaflets constituted flyers for jumble sales, tea parties, amateur drama and fundraising amusements of all sorts. These amusements were usually accommodated in the 'hall' or the library, where setting up and cleaning up could be factored into the total time input in achieving a successful day's takings at the door. Flag days noted in the *Irish Times* were very important opportunities to gather funds and inform the public. These amusements were conducted by teams of enthusiastic volunteers, often rallying the entire village into the project. Whether successful or not, everyone was thanked for their effort in the annual reports. In Dundrum, Milltown the Taney Players were regular contributors. Finally, there are some printed cards with the arrangements of the meetings of the association, indicating the time involved in organising the work and managing everything.[25]

The annual report for the year to the end of March 1967 does not indicate anything extraordinary except that the chairman, Mrs Mulvey, died suddenly. She had been a good friend to the nurses and her experience as an urban councillor was invaluable to the committee. A public health nurse had been appointed and was working well with the two Jubilee Nurses. Regretting the shortage of funds, they noted that many of the greatly increased population of Dundrum may not be aware of the service provided by the Jubilee nurses in the district. They also lamented the failure of fundraising efforts such as the planned fashion show for the Montrose Hotel which fell through.[26]

In September 1967 the committee received a distressing letter from Miss Quain, superintendent for the Queen's Institute. It was a call to an extraordinary general meeting, on 3rd October, in the Overend Hall, Leeson Street, Dublin.[27] The letter stated that there were difficulties recruiting nurses for training and that it was felt that the time had come to discontinue the service. It heralded the end of the Milltown, Dundrum District Nursing Association and many others around the country. Mrs J.M. Eyre, honorary secretary of the association, wrote on 29 September to the secretary of the Dublin Health Authority. The association presented its 53rd annual report and statement of accounts, giving notice that it was closing down as soon as possible. It left Naomi Overend and her committee with two major concerns, first, that nursing of elderly and patients would continue in their area and, second, that the nurses should receive full credit for their years of service and participate in pension arrangements at a later stage. The association offered to continue for a short period to facilitate a changeover. There were no more recorded letters.[28]

In 1936 the president, Lady Redmond, had stated in her report that 'as a voluntary institution the committee is in existence a considerable time and can look back upon the accomplishment of much useful work performed successfully and unostentatiously'.[29] This statement could equally have been made at the end. The service was closed down without the opportunity for even a little self-satisfaction on the part of the committee in the final report.

Dublin City Centre District Nursing Associations: St Patrick's and St Laurence's Training Homes

The training homes for Jubilee nurses, St Patrick's and St Laurence's, acted as the district nursing associations that provided a domiciliary service to much of Dublin city and its suburbs. There was a similar situation in Londonderry where the nursing students were supervised on the districts by the regular staff. Jubilee nurses did not carry out midwifery in Dublin as part of their training as the student nurses were already qualified midwives. Maternity care in those areas was provided by the Rotunda Hospital on the north side of the city and the National Maternity Hospital at Holles Street on the south. Inspections of the two Dublin homes were carried out by the superintendent of the Queen's Institute, Irish branch. Londonderry was inspected by the Queen's Institute in England. The number of staff varied throughout the period but in all three homes, through the early part of the twentieth century, there were usually five nursing staff and a supervisor for the ten or twelve students taken on every six months. The students lived in the home for their training until very much later in the scheme when the numbers were reduced. The six months spent in the poorest parts of Dublin, for many of the student nurses of all periods, seems to have left an everlasting impression on them.

Father Healy of Bray District Nursing Association

The *Irish Times* of 11 December 1895 reported a large meeting in the Shelbourne Hotel, Dublin in order to set up a cottage hospital in Bray, County Wicklow. Funds raised for the Father Healy Memorial, to the amount of £1,381, were not sufficient and it was decided to provide a district nurse instead.[30] Fr Healy, according to Elizabeth Countess of Fingall in her memoirs *Seventy Years Young*, was one of the many 'wits and storytellers' of Dublin. Describing the period of the Spencer viceroyalty 1882–1885, she remembered 'this famous Father Healy was still the simplest man alive, a good parish priest, much beloved by his parishioners, especially the poor'.[31] The Father Healy Memorial District Nursing Association was founded in 1896 for a population of 6,535. The secretary was

Miss Scott, with Mrs Meredith as president. Miss Scott was still secretary in 1935. By 1950 the secretary was Miss Hall of Árd na Gréine and the president was Aileen the Countess of Meath.[32] They decided to take fees as a means of financing their nurse and that they would not provide a midwifery service. The Father Healy Memorial District Nursing Association remained in existence until 1966.

The association's first nurse, Marion Batty, was transferred to Buncrana, County Donegal a year after the association was established. They hit the jackpot, however, with their second nurse, Josephine Purcell. Born in 1867 in Kanturk, County Cork, her father was a commissioned officer of the 91st Highlanders. She trained as a general nurse in Liverpool's Brownlow Hill Infirmary and as a Jubilee nurse in St Laurence's Home; she did not train as a midwife, as was common at that time. Beginning her first assignment at the Father Healy Memorial DNA, Bray in 1897, she took a short break due to illness in 1936 and died while still in their employ in 1937.[33] The inspector, Miss Michie, reported in 1920 that Josephine Purcell was a 'kind nurse, methods entirely out of date'; all other reports were satisfactory – not bad for 40 years of loyalty! The year after her death in 1938 a cottage was purchased by the committee. Anne Finucane came to them from Clane, County Kildare in 1937 and remained until 1950 when she left for home duties. She was replaced by Kathleen Logue, who qualified that year from St Patrick's Nurses Home. She was married in 1953 and re-joined as Mrs Maguire until the association's demise in 1966. Bray is a short train journey from Dublin and the Queen's inspectors usually attended the association's annual general meeting. In February 1966, the 'committee were adamant about closing down', according to Miss Delaney. They did so in May of that year.

Bray District Nursing Association

Bray is a large town on the coast, south of Dublin city. Two Queen's nurses, working concurrently, would have seemed logical for a district of its size, but this was only the case for a short period. Mrs Meredith, mentioned above, was named with Mrs Henry Kilshane in the setting up in 1908 of a Women's National Health

Association district nursing service in Bray. It was fully affiliated in 1910 for a greatly increased population of 10,000. It provided the fully furnished cottage from the beginning and the salary of the nurse was to be £90 p/a inclusive. The first nurse was Mary Josephine Hayes from St Laurence's Home. She left before the year was over, however, because the committee had sent her to London for further experience in connection with 'infant mortality work'. Henrietta O'Brien from Sutton TB, a Women's National Health Association home specialising in tuberculosis patients work, came for a year until the Bray association was temporarily closed. Katherine Dooley, who was not a Queen's Nurse, came in 1917 and stayed until 1929 when the association was, once again, disaffiliated.

Mallow District Nursing Association

Mallow, County Cork is a mid-sized town with a large hinterland. It had a district nursing association from 1895, known as the Mallow Nursing Society. Set up for a population of 4,439, its first honorary secretary was Mrs Purdon Coots. She resigned and was replaced by Mrs Webb of Wilton, Mallow. In 1950 Mrs Aubrey Thompson of Glenavon became secretary. The association did not provide midwifery in the beginning, and did not charge fees. Mrs William O'Brien remembers the Mallow Jubilee nurse in her book *My Irish Friends*. She relates that in a town where there were many divisions and dissentions, 'in all Mallow, Nurse [Emily] Gillespie had only friends'.[34] In her praise of the Jubilee nurse she describes her relationship as a committee member and friend. She also recounts their difficulties in trying to find suitable accommodation for the nurse.[35] In the early stages of the Queen's Institute most nurses stayed in lodgings where a landlady provided rooms and 'light attendance'. The rules of employment were very rigidly governed and two rooms were stipulated. It had been difficult to source accommodation and eventually the committee found a good woman to look after the nurse; however, the allocated sitting room was so full of ornaments it was ineffectual. It was in this cramped sitting room that the committee held its monthly meetings, 'where we decided the affairs of our little kingdom'.[36] The first Jubilee nurse in Mallow was Ellen Daly. She trained in St Laurence's Home and remained with Mallow for ten years, eventually leaving to take up a post as a senior nurse where she had trained. Sara Barry, who had trained as a Queen's nurse in Liverpool, replaced her. She stayed from 1898 to 1901, when she left to nurse privately. She was followed by the already-mentioned Emily Gillespie. It was her first district after training in St Laurence's Home in 1901. When she had to retire after 22 years because of ill health Mrs O'Brien describes the reaction of all the people of the town. 'One impulse seized the population, from the poorest to the richest. There were performances, plays and concerts to increase Nurse's fund. The result enabled her to retire in comfort to a little home by the sea.'[37] Nurse Gillespie was followed by Anna Clarke, who had come from Caherdaniel, County Kerry and only stayed for a year. Her successor, Kathleen McNamara, who had trained as a Queen's nurse in England, also only stayed for a year, leaving Mallow because of ill health. Ellen Connolly was next. She arrived from St Laurence's Home in 1925 and was transferred to Waterford in 1929. A newly qualified Annie O'Doherty was transferred to Bruckless, County Donegal after one year in Mallow. Nora Moloney then stayed for two years and took up a post as a public health nurse in 1930. Agnes Mary O'Reilly had just trained in St Laurence's in 1930 and stayed in Mallow until 1939 when she was transferred to Stillorgan, County Dublin. Finally Bridget Murphy came from Cahir, County Tipperary and remained, except for leave of absence due to ill health for six months in 1940, until she retired in 1962. During Nurse Murphy's period the association continued to experience accommodation problems, with the inspector noting in 1952 that accommodation was poor. In 1953 a new flat was secured. The nurse always received good reports but the committee was struggling with low funds towards the end. The association closed the year Nurse Murphy retired.

Ballinasloe District Nursing Association

The committee of the District Nursing Association, Ballinasloe, County Galway is an example of how a few strong people were able to get the whole town involved and excited by a single cause. A short-lived district nursing association was set up in 1908 under the auspices of the WNHA employing Nurse Maude Rutledge until it folded in 1911. In 1939 a new committee was set up with the parish priest, the Rev. E. Hughes, as president and Mrs Maureen Crohan, the Bank of Ireland manager's wife, as treasurer. They were fortunate to have as secretary Mrs Kathleen Kilduff, who may have known the previous committee as she was a national school teacher, from 1910, in Ballinasloe before her marriage.[38] The committee, which had a 'no fees' policy, was made up of eight to ten representatives from all sectors of the community in Ballinasloe and the surrounding countryside. It included the already-mentioned bank manager's wife, a teacher in the national school, the wife of the owner of a public house in the town, a lady who ran the newsagent's and the wife of the local solicitor. Mrs Kilduff ran the committee, as her son described her, as 'commander and chief' until its dissolution in 1955. Mrs Kilduff was married to the town harness-maker, in the days before cars and tractors became the norm, this was a vital and busy profession. She held regular meetings of the Ballinasloe District Nursing Association in her large kitchen; sandwiches were made and business was conducted as required. Meetings were held before and after the annual door-to-door collections to count and record the donations. The committee would meet to organise the bi-annual jumble sales, a vital part of fundraising and of redistribution of goods, particularly clothes, in times of extreme hardship. Finally, there would be several meetings to discuss the annual highlight of Ballinasloe's social calendar, the 'Nurses' Dance'. Rory, Mrs Kilduff's son, remembers being part of the team decorating the Town Hall for the event. He said it was vital to hire a good band such as 'Stephen Garvey' and that the 3/- 6d ticket included supper.[39] In 1945 the nurse's dance raised £63, which was a considerable part of the association's income. The association collected £87. 15/- 16d on door-to-door collections that year. In January 1950 Mrs Kilduff had written to the Maternity and Child Welfare Recoupment Claims Department in the Custom House in Dublin asking if the tax paid on expenses for the dance could be reclaimed.[40] Mr Kilduff said that people liked, if possible, to give a donation to the nurse because it gave them a feeling of importance. Unlike many of the nursing committees, towards the end of the period, Ballinasloe

District Nursing Association still had money in the bank, and £167 was given to the local parish priest for a suitable charity. The association had employed Nurse Mary Agnes O'Grady, newly qualified from St Patrick's Nurses Home, from 1936 for twenty years until her death, following an operation, in 1955. The committee rented a centrally located, comfortable cottage and provided fuel for Nurse O'Grady. In 1939 the inspector, Miss Burke, noted that the nurse was living in a new cottage. As a respected member of the community she was a regular visitor to Mrs Kilduff's for evening tea. A neighbour of Nurse O'Grady, Mr Mathew Ganly, remembers that she knew and was appreciated by everyone in the parish and was a vital assistant to the dispensary doctor.[41] Nurse O'Grady was not expected to do midwifery cases because there was a dispensary midwife in the town and Portiuncula Hospital opened in 1945, but her neighbour says she was occasionally called to emergency cases when needed.[42]

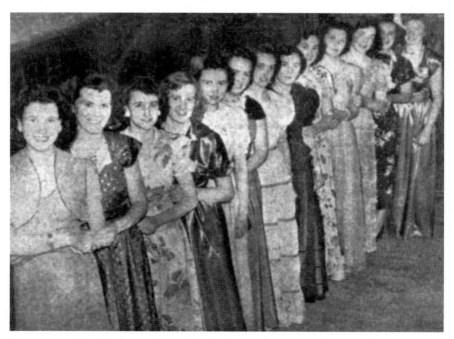

The Cavan Jubilee Nurses' Dance. Great organisation, a good band and months of dressmaking for the annual nurses' dance guaranteed a good night for all.
Courtesy of Dr Áine Sullivan.

Naas District Nursing Association

Naas, County Kildare began a voluntary district nursing service in 1895 for a population of 3,808. It lasted 72 years. It was set up by the Countess of Mayo, who was the president, with Lady Albreda Bourke as chairwoman. The honourable secretaries were, first, Miss P. O'Farrell and later Mrs H. Farrell. Mrs Browne of Abbeyfield was in charge in the 1930s and was superseded by Miss de Burgh of ÁrdCuin. The association applied for a grant of £20 per annum for TB work. It did not offer a midwifery service initially, and did not charge fees to patients.

Naas District Nursing Association began in the early stages by offering the nurse board, which was costing the association 10/- per week, and lodging with attendance which was £25 per annum. Laundry was 2/- per month. The nurse's salary was £30 per annum, to rise to £35. In 1905 a furnished house was provided for the nurse, and by 1918 the salary had increased to £100 inclusive. The first nurse was Alice Walshe, who had come from Drogheda, County Louth and was eventually transferred in 1903. Gertrude Chapman and Marion Laughney stayed a year each before being transferred to other districts. Lucy McColther came from Galway and stayed until 1907 when she resigned. Mary Lee, newly trained, stayed until 1913, and her successor Josephine McNulty was married in 1915. Louise Shaw came back from active service and left the same year for other work. Elizabeth Ross came from Achill Island, County Mayo and left again in 1916 for active service. Aileen Mooney stayed for three years before leaving on sick leave in 1919. The newly qualified Mary Kate McKelvey joined for six years before leaving for other work. Alice Maude Hanrahan went to the US in 1928. She was replaced by Lilly Tipping for a year. Cecilia Dillon came from Rosmuck, County Galway in 1929. She was ill for some months in 1940, when a temporary nurse was appointed, but remained in the district until 1963.

In 1950 the Queen's inspector Miss Aylward had a strong disagreement with the secretary of the committee because the house for the nurse was not suitable. There was a second inspection that year but at that point the house issue remained unresolved. It must have been sorted at some stage, but in 1957 Nurse Dillon was finding the work very heavy. She was ill in 1960 and the committee was having financial problems, but once again seemed to have pulled through. Nurse Dillon retired in 1963 on a pension after 34 years' service to the community of Naas and its surrounding area. There were a series of nurses, including Theresa McGrainey who stayed for two years and four other nurses, each staying about a year. One of these was Catherine Mary McGuinness, who had recently come from St Patrick's Home and left to take up a public health post. We interviewed her as Mrs Mary Byrne and her contribution to Chapter 1 ('Queen's Nurse') is invaluable. The inspector said of Nurse McGuinness that she had 'made a good impression and has plenty of work'. This is not surprising as Naas was a rapidly expanding town at the time.

Mr Liam Kenny of Naas wrote informing us of a treasure trove of material that was contemporary with the District Nursing Association. The *Kildare Observer* has an online archive covering the period 1880 to 1935 courtesy of Kildare County Council, the British Library and National Micro Media Ltd. This archive gives an invaluable insight into the workings of an average district nursing association over a short period of time. It comprises advertisements and reports relating to the committee, nurse and nursing matters. Many monthly meetings of the early Naas District Nursing Association were reported in this local paper. It began with everyday matters such as the payment of the nurse's salary cheque being signed. This became repetitive after a few years. The reports also focused on fundraising efforts, such as the proceeds of the Naas Cricket Club's benefit match being donated to the association with half the proceeds to go to the nurse, as a bonus, in 1918. As the association became more established, reporting of monthly meetings was less frequent, with only important issues, such as resolutions, being recorded. The Countess of Mayo, president of the association, was very involved and attended most months. She and Mrs J. Rorke signed the following resolution on 20 October 1928:

> We feel that in addition to the subsidy which is paid by the Naas Urban Council to the District Nursing Association for the services of the nurse in their maternity and child welfare scheme, some provision ought to be made for the supply of milk to infants and nursing mothers.[43]

This resolution was to be sent by Mrs Farrell, the honorary secretary, to all the respective funding boards. The newspaper included small classified advertisements, such as the one on 15 October 1910 for 'Strong Narcissus Bulbs', of many varieties, 4d for a dozen. They were available from Miss Culshaw, of Johnstown Inn, for the benefit of Naas District Nursing Association.

The Naas DNA relied for extra funding, like many of its peers, on the 'dance' held usually in the Town Hall in February. It was very well advertised and in 1931 the association had Manahan's Band (personally conducted). The dance committee provided supper with the assistance of Mrs Lawlor. A single ticket cost 10/- and a double 17/- 6d, which you could purchase from any member of the committee or at the door.[44] On 9 April 1927 the committee began publicising a choral concert and plays. These were to be presented by Naas Choral and Dramatic Union in Naas Town Hall over the weekend beginning Friday, 22 April 1927. People were encouraged to 'Support generously a generous performance for a great charity'.[45]

There was an interesting article in 1930 titled 'Health Conditions in County Kildare'. It was an extract from the annual report of the County Kildare Medical Officer. It said there were eleven district nursing associations in the county and discussed their involvement with attempts to reduce infant mortality. Kildare was a significantly rural county at the time. It was believed that the 'assistance and advice of the nurse can do much to reduce maternal mortality and conserve infant life'. Miss Colburn, superintendent of the Queen's Institute, was running a course to advise nurses on post-natal care. All the nurses from Kildare were instructed to attend. Mothers of weak infants were encouraged away from the fatalist view of their babies' wellbeing to seek medical assistance wherever available. The medical officer reported extraordinary success with this programme: 'The number of deaths of infants under one year of age has fallen from 101 in 1929 to 65 in 1930.'[46]

All district nursing associations, dependent on voluntary effort, refined the skill of thank you. Local papers such as the *Kildare Observer* were useful in this regard. A letter to the editor in the Saturday edition of 23 February 1929 began:

> Sir, will you allow us through your columns to express our gratitude to all those who by gifts, loans and personal service enabled the committee … to carry the dance to such a successful issue.

The association was expressing its thanks to all those who helped with a fundraiser for the district nurse's pension fund, at which £84 was raised after expenses.[47]

Portmarnock, Balgriffin, Baldoyle and Kinsealy District Nursing Association, County Dublin

This coastal region on the north side of Dublin has a large rural catchment area. A district nursing association was founded in 1898 and was affiliated in 1899. The first secretary was Mrs Symes, Lime Hill, Raheny. The association provided two rooms, fire, light and attendance for the nurse. There was to be no midwifery offered and no fees were to be charged to the patients. In its 68 years' existence the association employed ten nurses. The last was Mary Kenny; she began in 1937 and was married in 1953. She continued, as Mrs Harrington, in the district until the end of the scheme in 1966.

By 1949 the association had become Portmarnock, Baldoyle and District Queen's District Nursing Association. That year, it abandoned the Samaritan fund and was worried that subscriptions had not increased while expenses had. The association was also concerned that it may no longer be able to support Nurse Kenny. She had 358 general nursing cases, to whom she had paid 3,936 visits. There were 214 children under five and they required 2,319 visits. Some 176 mothers were called upon 1,518 times. There were 27 patients with TB in the district that year, to whom 714 calls were made.[48]

Mrs Kennedy was interviewed in her home in Malahide about her time as secretary of Portmarnock District Nursing Association and as a member of the council of the Queen's Institute in later years. She said she was contacted when she was expecting her first baby and joined after the baby was born. As a qualified doctor she was, like many of her peers, prevented from continuing her career due to the marriage bar. For her personally it was important to choose a charity project that was not associated with any church organisation. The value of the Jubilee nurses was that they kept the old people independent, and in their own homes, for longer. The district had a mature population at the time with few new residents and babies. This meant the nurse did not have a huge responsibility in terms of child welfare. Mrs Kennedy was secretary of the association from 1950. She replaced the first secretary, Mrs Symes, who had set up the district. She was also involved in the St John Ambulance and the Multiple Sclerosis Society. She said charity work helped to give one a social outlet and people had the time in those days. Her family lived on the north side of the city, where the training home for nurses was Catholic, and the people thought the name Jubilee nurse celebrated the pope's jubilee. Funding was mostly door to door; usually you got a 6d coin and once she nearly fell off a doorstep because she was handed a pound note. There was always the Christmas raffle and those dreadful jumble sales. They met once a month in committee members' houses, her own sometimes, or the home of Mrs Pringle. The committee included the school mistress and farmers' wives from the area. Mrs Kennedy remembers meeting in the mornings and having coffee afterwards. It was very efficiently run; there was no waste. She said there was a lot of work but it was very satisfying to achieve something. The nurse never wanted a car and was happy enough to cycle around the district. She also had her own home after her marriage, which was an advantage for the committee. When asked about the garden scheme she said her mother in law opened her garden for a day. Afterwards there was pandemonium because it was discovered that a rose bush had been pinched! Like other districts, at the end of the scheme the committee went on to visit and look after the interests of the older people in the community.

Birr District Nursing Association

In 1905 Cassandra the Countess of Rosse, wife of the fourth Earl, called for the setting up of Birr Jubilee Nursing Association. She provided furnished lodgings, fire, light and attendance for the nurse. She became its president and the vice-presidents were jointly the parish priest, the rector and the Methodist minister. Birr is a medium-sized town in the very centre of Ireland with a large rural hinterland in what was then King's County (County Offaly). The population of the district was 4,400. The usual preliminary inspection was carried out in 1905 by Miss Lamont.

Anne the Countess of Rosse, married to the sixth Earl, took over the presidency from her grandmother–in-law in 1936. She remained in the position until the association ceased operations in 1971.

The first secretary, appointed in 1906, was Miss Anna Bennett. Her term ended in 1925 and she died the following year. Miss Alice Woods of Wilmer Terrace, Birr became secretary. She was from a medical family and had relevant knowledge and practical experience. The committee met in her honour shortly after her death in 1947 aged 94. Lady Rosse was unable to attend and sent a letter in which she said Miss Woods was much loved and appreciated and a very successful administrator of the association.[49] Mrs George Keele had helped Miss Woods as assistant secretary for a while. Following the death of Miss Woods in 1947 Mrs Kathleen Doolan of 7 Oxmantown Mall, Birr took over the post of honourable secretary.[50] She remained as honourable secretary until 1971.

Mrs Jamie Power was the first treasurer, from 1906 to 1926. Mrs K.F. Barry stayed for a few months and was followed by Mrs J.A. Dooley until 1928. The post was then filled by Miss M. Dooley until 1939 and she was followed by Mrs Marie Barry until 1945. Finally Mrs O'Donohoe took on the onerous responsibility of ensuring that every hard-won penny of the money collected was used correctly.

In 1918 the nurse's salary was £85. 10/- 3d and her rent was free. In 1921 the salary was increased to £123. 10/-, which included her rooms. In 1945 the salary was £194. 10/- plus rent and travelling expenses. The Queen's Institute did not record if midwifery was taken, but the association did not apply for the child welfare grant; only the TB grant of £50 was mentioned on the year of setting up. We know that in 1956 the district nursing association decided to take a grant for midwifery and lost its nurse the following year because of it. The first nurse sent to Birr district, Margaret Kerr, was newly qualified from St Laurence's Home. She left after two years to do further studies in Alexandra College. When she was leaving Birr, the urban council officially recognised that

> … she won the universal admiration and gratitude of all with whom she was brought in contact … In the noble profession she adorned

she displayed the highest proficiency, and combined an urbanity of manner, kindliness of disposition, and untiring zeal with an attention worthy of the highest commendation.[51]

Margaret Kerr was followed by Mary J. Dalton in 1908, again a graduate of St Laurence's. She stayed until 1920, when she had to leave because of marriage. Mary O'Neill came for two years and left because of ill health. A temporary Queen's nurse, Ellen Walshe, arrived in 1922 and was eventually transferred to Waterford in 1926. The nurse who succeeded her came from Waterford and stayed until she too had to leave for marriage in 1933. Geraldine Bridget Fitzgerald was transferred to Dublin after twelve years. She had been newly qualified from St Laurence's Home in 1933 and left in 1945. A letter signed by all on the committee outlined how 'it would be difficult to convey to you how much your departure is regretted, not only by the committee, but quite as much by the innumerable patients you nursed with such patience, skill and kindness during the twelve years you spent in Birr'. On presentation of a parting gift, Miss Fitzgerald was told that 'if the good wishes accompanying this gift could add to its intrinsic value it would indeed be priceless'.[52] This committee was also adept at thanking people; as mentioned already, it is essential for any organisation relying primarily on voluntary workers to raise funds. Mary E. O'Hara, who succeeded Nurse Fitzgerald, only stayed a few months and left for home reasons. The next two nurses, Mary Ellen Monaghan and Mary Theresa Killian, both left to do public health district nursing work. Nurse Monaghan came from Castlecomer, County Monaghan and stayed from 1946 to 1952. During her stay a new nurse's house was organised in 1949. Nurse Killian came from Clonmel, County Tipperary and only stayed for a year. Angela O'Rourke, who succeeded her, came from the Lady Dudley district of Lettermullan, County Galway in 1953.

In 1956 Miss Aylward, the Queen's inspector, noted that the funds were very low, and the committee was asked by the local council to take on midwifery work.[53] Nurse O'Rourke asked for a transfer, and left in 1958. The last Queen's nurse to work for Birr DNA was Margaret McEvoy from Mountmellick, County Laois, the daughter of a retired sergeant in the Royal Irish Constabulary. She trained as a general nurse in London and in Lancashire as a midwife. She qualified from St Patrick's Home in July 1948 and her first district was Tully, Spiddal, County Galway for a year, followed by Multifarnham, County Westmeath for four years. She was transferred to Clane, County Kildare and remained another four years before coming to Birr. She remained from 1958 until 1971, when the district finally closed. All reports on Nurse McEvoy were positive; she was 'liked by her committee and was a kind popular nurse'.[54]

The present Earl and Countess of Rosse allowed us to view a comprehensive collection of documents relating to Birr Jubilee Nursing Association. Assembled by Lord Rosse's mother and great-grandmother, it contains letters and documents relating to the association's beginnings in 1905. Documents were still collected presenting the predicament the committee found itself in when organising further employment for nurse McEvoy in 1971. Minutes of meetings and official communications from the Queen's Institute and the county council were in the same envelope as newspaper cuttings, handwritten notes on fundraisers, meetings, lunches and well-wishes. The collection illustrates the very time-consuming, often perturbing and very social aspects of running an efficient and successful district nursing association.

Apart from the already-noted tendency of families to pass this voluntary work on to the next generation, the remarkable element of the collection is Mrs Doolan. Evidence of her energy and commitment is everywhere. She and Lady Rosse worked closely on the association and she was an 'inspiring friend' according to the Countess of Rosse in an obituary she wrote for Mrs Doolan in 1984. She 'gave her life and energy to the cause of the Jubilee Nursing Association in Birr; second-best would never do for anything she undertook'.[55] As secretary of the Jubilee Nursing Association from before 1946 until it closed in 1971, her work was practically full time and absolutely unpaid. It was Mrs Doolan who listened to the nurses and their problems and mediated arrangements that would suit all. She wrote countless letters, agendas and minutes, organised and attended all the meetings, fundraisers and parties. She was in constant contact with the members of the association, particularly those on the committee. It was especially important to ensure that the money collectors and fundraising event managers were met regularly.

One of the committee members, Mrs Kathleen McEvoy, known in that period as Mrs Joe Kennedy, contacted us to relate her experiences as a member of the committee. She had been on the committee from 1949 to 1971 when it closed. She was a neighbour of Mrs Doolan. As the wife of the dentist she said that the people on the committee were all from professional backgrounds, not business, except Mr Woods who was a manufacturer in the town. She also said that all of the clergymen in the town attended the monthly meetings as they were on the committee. She remembered the meetings were held in Birr Castle and afternoon tea was served later. The nurse usually came to the meetings. She said if the countess was unable to attend, the chair was taken by a rather elderly lady who was the widow of a banker. She remembers discussions on the organisation of the endless fundraisers, including the whist drives, the garden fêtes in the castle, and a bazaar and cake sale in Dooley's Hotel. Lady Rosse would send the chauffeur to collect boxes of stuff for the jumble sale.

Mrs Doolan's work as secretary was to coordinate everyone involved. She communicated with doctors, the county council, the Queen's Institute and regularly reported in beautiful handwritten letters to Lady Rosse, who seemed to be away a lot. These letters give an insight into the daily worries – and triumphs – that they encountered. On 27 June 1948, following a very successful visit of the Queen's inspector Miss Kenny, Mrs Doolan wrote to Lady Rosse. She enclosed a very healthy balance sheet and said that their funds were secure, adding that the government would not be taking over anytime soon. This was two years after the Public Health Bill which threatened to remove all subsidies and, in effect, close all district nursing associations.

Another letter from Mrs Doolan to Lady Rosse dated 6 December 1956 read:

Dear Lady Rosse,

At last I got the jumble sale figures – I hope. Only last night I got £2-balance of Mrs Haslam's sales. Money has been coming in in 'dribs and drabs' since the sale, and what a nuisance. They were all more eager to buy than last year but, as Mrs Drought remarked, we had to fight a hard battle for every penny. Already I am deluged with reminders for

Christmas. We are having the meeting re benefits on next Wednesday. I had a visit from Miss Delaney Inspector today. She was very pleased with everything and said that every home she visited with nurse the patients were all full of praise. There has been no communication from Dr Reeves since and Miss Delaney told me the office in Dublin has had no communication from him. The petrol shortage is causing great inconvenience and much unemployment. It must be worse in England. You will see by the balance sheet that our profits are £14-19-2 more than last year. Extraordinary considering everyone is feeling gloomy. Let's hope now that we can give a little help where most needed.

All good wishes
Yours sincerely
Kathleen Doolan

The reference to Dr Reeves, the County Medical Officer of Health, was that he suggested to Miss Delaney of the Queen's Institute that the Jubilee nurse in Birr take midwifery duties. Nurse O'Rourke was not happy about the suggestion and her transfer was in question. As mentioned above, Nurse O'Rourke lost the battle and was replaced by Nurse McEvoy.

A series of letters began on 27 November 1967 with regard to the closing down of the association and the re-employment of the nurse. The first letter was from Dr A. Reeves to Nurse McEvoy. It suggests that there would be no problem for Nurse McEvoy to become a public health nurse in her area, 'as the Minister has indicated his willingness to approve of the appointment in certain cases'.[56] Jubilee nurses were highly qualified and already established in their areas as the primary community nurses, but civil servants did not accept their status automatically. Mrs Doolan wrote to Lady Rosse enclosing a copy of the letter, saying with relief 'our days are numbered'. The association continued to operate as usual without the support of the Queen's Institute because Nurse McEvoy's employment, despite the above letter, was still not secure. In September 1970 they received a letter from Offaly County Council saying that it would employ the nurse through the health authority but that the district nursing association would still be the employer. The letter included a long list of stipulations that the committee was not sure it could meet. Mrs Doolan, in a letter to Lady Rosse, shows her exasperation: 'The accompanying letter should solve our problems, or does it?' In October that year the county council said it would not accept responsibility for the nurse's full salary but would continue to pay a subsidy. They were back at square one. The Queen's Institute had closed in 1967 and Birr District Nursing Association could not afford to continue without support for much longer. At last, in December 1970, Lady Rosse received a letter from the Department of Health stating that Miss McEvoy would be fully employed by Offaly County Council, taking with her pension entitlements, once she had filled in the requisite paperwork. The committee of Birr District Nursing Association, in a reception at Birr Castle and with great fanfare in the *Midland Tribune*, handed over to the County Manager in February 1971.[57]

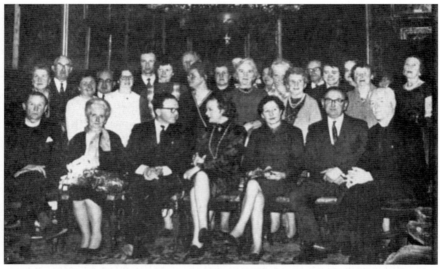

Birr District Nursing Association handing over to the county council in February 1971. Front row, L to R – Rev F.R. Bourke, Rector (Vice-President); Mrs M..J. Doolan (Hon. Sec.); Mr P. Dowd (Laois-Offaly County Manager); The Countess of Rosse (President); Nurse Margaret McEvoy; Mr W. Haslam (Chairman of Birr UDC); Rev Msgr P.J. Hamell P.P. (Vice-President).
Courtesy of the *Midland Tribune*, Birr.

Newtowncunningham, Burt and Killea Nursing Association

One of the later district nursing associations to be affiliated was Newtowncunningham, Burt and Killea, County Donegal, in 1950. This rural district is situated on the picturesque Derry side of Lough Swilly, not far from Letterkenny. A Jubilee nurse was proposed by a female Dr Waggott in September 1945 but the nurse only arrived in 1951. In 1946 a letter to the 520 members apologises for the delay and blames the new Public Health Bill, to be passed in the Dáil and Seanad before district nursing associations would know if they were permitted to continue. The committee at that time was to comprise Mrs F. Bowen as president and Mr H. Diver as secretary. The names recorded in the Queen's Institute as the official committee, however, were Major Power of Mason Lodge, Newtowncunningham as president and Mr H. Diver, Moness, Burt as secretary. Treasurers were Mrs J. Maguire, Miss T. Surpless, a national school teacher in Burt, and Mrs R.W. Cunningham of the Moyle, Newtowncunningham.[58] By the time of the first annual report, and Miss Greene the nurse had completed a year's work, the new president was Dr W.K. Bigger of Bogay House, Newtowncunningham and the secretary was Mr H. Diver. This was February 1952 and a new committee, with a balance based on the different parishes, was proposed. Long lists of collectors were already well established and this appears to be the main means of funding chosen by the committee. In March of that year at a public meeting in the Columban Hall, Newtowncunningham a new list of members was elected and Mrs Chance's name appears for the first time. The records kept by this association include the handwritten minutes, on four small hardback copies, from the very beginning to its end in 1974. They recorded the years 1945–1956, 1956–1964, 1964–1971 and an incomplete book from 1971–1974. Rev. Fr Muldoon, CC, the last chairman of the association, asked at the final meeting that the minute books be kept. They give a very human side to this history. These copybooks show people puzzling and sorting out, as they go along, the day-to-day difficulties of administrating a voluntary organisation. An assembly of papers and notes are also in the archives. They include occasional printed annual reports, letters and many financial statements. These are now accessible in the Donegal Archives in Lifford.[59]

The minutes from February 1951, before the nurse took up her duties, detailed that her services would be free and that if patients gave a donation to her these would go to the funds of the association. 'There was a very considerable search for accommodation for the nurse, it was not ideal, but she had her own furnished sitting room. furnished bedroom, the use of the kitchen and also a small kitchen of her own.'[60] These were the exact specifications of the Queen's Institute. Dr White, the dispensary doctor for this and other districts in the area, said that medical supplies would be covered by the expenses of his dispensary. He congratulated the committee on its good control of the finances. Parish priest Fr Carr and Rev. Mr Parker would both use their pulpits to interest the public in the scheme. They felt that once the nurse began her work it would speak for itself.

Mrs Marguerite (or Peg) Chance was appointed secretary officially in February 1955 on the resignation of Miss T. Surpless. Mrs Chance's mother-in-law was Lady Eileen Chance, who was on the committee of the Queen's Institute in Dublin around the period 1924–1930. Her brother-in-law, Mr Leslie Chance, an accountant, was invited to be a member of the Queen's Institute in 1965.[61] Peg Chance's very distinctive handwriting was very rarely missing from the books following her appointment as secretary in 1955. She was the core manager for the association until it closed nineteen years later. She would have been aware of the Queen's nurses of her childhood in Wales. She and her husband, who grew up in Milltown, County Dublin, came to Donegal in 1949.[62]

There were six nurses employed in the period. They were, as previously mentioned, Miss Greene who was newly qualified from St Patrick's Home and left in 1952 for 'home duties'; Frances Hogan, who arrived also from St Patrick's and stayed for two years before being transferred to Rathcoole, County Dublin; Ann McGovern, who arrived from Lettermullan, County Galway and was transferred to Portlaw, County Waterford in 1957; Margaret McCauley, who started in 1957 and retired in 1968 on a pension; Lily Anne Curran, who came from St Patrick's Home in 1964 and left in 1966 for public health work;[63] and Mrs Duffy, who had worked initially in Taughboyne, County Donegal and helped out from time to time with holidays and relief assistance. Mrs Duffy came as a temporary nurse in January 1966 and stayed on until they closed in 1974. She then became the public health nurse for the area until she retired. We interviewed Mary Duffy and her outstanding story is featured in Chapter 1.

Committee meetings were held monthly, or as required, in the Columban Hall in Newtowncunningham. Dr Bigger was usually the chairman, and in his absence Rev. Parker presided. Meetings were usually attended by the nurse, and the minutes included her report and often the sending of a letter of sympathy to members on bereavements. Printed stationery was used and had to be ordered from time to time. The annual general meeting had to be arranged. When the Queen's inspector, and very occasionally the superintendent, came from Dublin it was recorded, as was the inspector's report, which always followed the visit. Over the years the nurse's accommodation took up a great deal of the committee's time, as finding suitable rooms could be problematic, and what would suit one nurse may not be appropriate for another. It was very important that the nurse live in the centre of a very large district, so that everyone subscribing would be aware of her comings and goings. This was more practical too as the nurse had less distance to cover on her bicycle. In the later stages the acquisition of a site and efforts to get the local council to build a suitable house became a preoccupation. When Mrs Duffy came she had her own home and car. This district was very large, hilly and with a scattered population so the committee came up with a rather novel way to overcome the problem. They stated in their printed annual report for the year ending 1952: 'Car owners in the district were therefore asked to assist in transporting the nurse. The response was sufficient to provide transport on two mornings a week during the winter months and it is hoped that it will be possible to increase this service next winter.'[64] The arrangement was praised by the Queen's Institute in its report letters. The minutes often included the names of new people who it was suggested might help in this commitment, which was, of course, coordinated by Mrs Chance.[65] In 1957 the new nurse McCauley found her bicycle too heavy, despite the fact that the association's transport scheme in March 1956 was 'going satisfactorily'.[66] Discussion of this in a group interview in the home of Mr Michael Chance, son of Mrs Chance the secretary, was interesting. It appears that being a driver for the nurse was not seen as a drudge obligation and was carried out mostly by farmers' wives in the area, who thoroughly enjoyed being out with the nurse.[67]

From the very beginning it was decided that collections were to be the primary source of funding,[68] as was the case with most of the Donegal and rural district nursing associations or health clubs. The Jubilee nurse in the area was called the 'penny nurse' according to the members of the association who were interviewed. Collection was not a problem. People kept their contribution aside and never questioned the fact that the government had, for several years, taken over almost every other district. There was a deep appreciation for the work the nurse did in the community and a personal affection for her.[69] A book was issued to each collection area with a list of all householders. The success or otherwise of door to door collections was discussed at committee meetings. Occasional comments were noted from the subscribers, such as that they felt they did not see the nurse enough in their area. The finances of this district nursing association were usually very good, and the committee was congratulated by the Queen's inspector from time to time. Grants were applied for and received, like most of the other district nursing associations around the country. The other main means of fundraising was the Nursing Association Dance. Arrangements for the dance, to be held in November or December in Burt Hall, began in January. Picking a date that did not clash with any other event, and also early booking of a good band, was vital. A sub-committee in charge of the dance, later in the year, would meet in Dr Bigger's house. Then the fine detail would be worked out, such as food for the supper, spot prizes, cloakroom attendants, decorating the hall, printed posters in public places, press notifications and invitations to the local dignitaries.[70] The dance was, according to the ladies interviewed in Mr Chance's house, the highlight of the year. It was very expensive at 10/- for the ticket but worth every penny.[71]

In May 1968 a letter was sent, with the annual report, to all subscribers informing them of the decision of the Queen's Institute to close down. The letter added: 'We are in the happy position of having an excellent nurse we are able to carry on provided we have your continued support.'[72] The association did continue to get the support it needed for almost six more years. The minutes of the last meeting of the association on 25 March 1974 discussed closing on 4 April of that year. The reason seemed to be that 'The eight Lady Dudley nurses were going over to public health and Convoy were also closing shortly'. Convoy was another district nursing association in the Donegal region. Mrs Duffy was to be employed as public health nurse and was eligible for superannuation. A letter of thanks was to be sent to all collectors and the closing down notice put in the press. The association still had money in the bank and proposed giving it to a fund for the aged. Peg Chance was honourable secretary of the Newtowncunningham Care of the Aged Committee, which evolved from the district nursing association. A handwritten memo in 1974 noted that the actual expenditure for the association in 1952, the first full year of employing a nurse, was £360. 10/- 00 and by 1974 it was £2559.81. Mrs Chance continued to contact nurses from all over Donegal for many years, and her son remembers visiting retired and working nurses during 'days out' over this period.

Taughboyne District Nursing Association

More commonly known today as Carrigens, this was a neighbouring district of Newtowncunningham, County Donegal but closer to Derry. The association was founded in 1941 by its president, Fr Johnstone and secretary, Ms J.K. Baird, of Duncally, Carrigens. Mrs Baird remained secretary until its closure in 1967.

The first nurse employed in Taughboyne was Jane Roberts Davis, who transferred to Northern Ireland in 1943. Bridget Loughney stayed five years before she left to get married and Mary Kearns was there for three years before she also got married. Mary Kearns came back to work as the last nurse in Newtowncunningham, Burt and Killea as Mrs Duffy and is an important contributor to our chapter on the Queen's Nurse (Chapter 1). When she left, Kathleen McConigley came from Dundrum District Nursing Association, County Dublin and stayed for three years before accepting a position with a hospital. Sara McKeown stayed for three years before her marriage in 1958. Catherine Prior was transferred to Newtownmountkennedy, County Wicklow after a year and Christina Hannon spent a year also in Taughboyne before going to the US. Rose O'Reilly was with the association for one year until Mrs Pearson arrived as a temporary Queen's nurse. Mrs Pearson is also one of our featured nurses in Chapter 4 and she remained with

Taughboyne DNA until its closure in 1967. Following the association's demise, she says, the committee continued to support local voluntary causes.[73]

Manorcunningham District Nursing Association

In the same area as the other two districts mentioned above but nearer to Letterkenny was Manorcunningham DNA, County Donegal. A legacy of £800 was left in 1941 by Miss Davis 'to provide a Jubilee nurse for this area'. The honorary secretary was Mrs Mary Bradley, Manorcunningham, while the treasurer was Mrs McNulty of Gort. They had found suitable lodgings for a nurse, two good rooms separate from the household. Miss Kavanagh the inspector complimented them on a solid beginning.

The first nurse in Manorcunningham was Mary Shovlin from St Patrick's Home. She stayed until 1945 when she was transferred to Clonmany, County Donegal. Catherine Sweeney came from Castlecomer, County Kilkenny and stayed one year before moving to Ramelton, County Donegal. Kate Quinn stayed two years, before being transferred to Castlerea, County Roscommon. Bridget Brennan only stayed one year until 1949, a year in which the association seems to have encountered a spot of bother. According to the inspector, the 'nurse was unsettled and the committee seem to have lost interest'. The association appears to have reopened in 1966 when a Mrs Singleton re-joined. We do not have details of when it finally closed.

Dalkey, Killiney and Ballybrack District Nursing Association

Comprising a very pretty seaside district of three small villages close to Dublin city with good public transport, this association was the eighth district nursing association registered with the Queen's Institute. Set up in 1893 for a population of 3,234 people, it was one of the longest surviving association in the country, closing in 1966. The committee decided to provide midwifery and not to charge fees. The first secretary was Miss Synnott, Innismore, Glenageary, County Dublin. She was replaced by Miss Ivy and then Miss Muster, both of whom resigned. The last named honorary secretary was Mrs Sherlock, Summerfield, Dalkey. She was still the secretary in 1935. The association received a grant from the Queen's Institute of £20 to set up, and the first nurse had furnished rooms and a salary of £35. 36/-, with uniform also provided. The last nurses were Mrs Hogan from 1957 and Miss Tubridy, who had trained in St Patrick's, and started with the association in 1961. The history of this association shows a strong committee as there was a lot of coming and going of nurses over the 73 years. Eighteen nurses worked in the district, although if the Queen's inspector did not record nurses' maiden names on the register it is hard to tell whether some of those who were married joined again. Four of the nurses over the years left the association to become public health nurses. The first few nurses only lasted a year or less and in 1902 Kathleen Blake arrived. She did not appear to have good health and had to take leave of absence in the winter months a few times, leaving eventually in 1921 due to ill health. Her replacement, Elizabeth McNally, came from the district nursing association in Tralee, County Kerry and remained for five years. In 1928 another nurse with health issues arrived. She was Mary Reynolds and had to take sick leave for an unspecified period in 1933. She again took a period of absence from the district in 1935 for home duties (this often meant taking care of elderly parents but is rarely specified), finally leaving in 1940. While these nurses were on leave a series of temporary nurses were sent from the institute and a second nurse was hired to assist Nurse Reynolds. Two nurses were employed from that period on. Mary Durkin trained in St Laurence's Home in 1940. This was her first district and she stayed until 1949 before accepting a public health post. Margaret Breen, who had been a temporary nurse in 1935, was employed as Mrs McGinley in 1950 until 1953. Mary Morkler had been with the association from 1955 as a newly trained Jubilee nurse from St Patrick's Home and left for marriage in 1961. In 1955 Miss Delaney, the Queen's inspector, reported that a new house was provided for both nurses together. She also noted that the funds of the district nursing association were low, but this seemed to have been sorted out, as it did not close for another eleven years.

Later committee members were rarely recorded on the Queen's list of affiliated districts. An interview with two committee members, Mrs Joan Hall and Mrs Anne Purcell, conducted in the home of Mrs Hall on 20 July 2011, gave a very good insight into the workings of this urban district nursing association. Mrs Hall says she joined the committee in 1950 on the death of her mother, who had also been on the committee. She was treasurer at first, taking a break for a few months when her baby was born. She does not remember paying salaries, which was probably the job of the secretary or chairwoman. This task was more than likely carried out by Mrs Molly Conan, described by Mrs Hall as the 'top and tail' of the organisation until her death, when Mrs Cynthia Fitzpatrick took over. Mrs Fitzpatrick was the wife of the local doctor in private practice, as distinct from the dispensary doctor. The committee seemed to operate without designated titles. Mrs Hall said that, as in many situations in life, there was a core of two or three people who did all the work. She remembered Miss Muriel McComas as a very active and hard-working member of the committee, probably secretary. Mrs Freda Hurley was possibly secretary or treasurer at different times. It was very difficult, it seems, to say no to Mrs Conan, a very good attribute for the main organiser of a voluntary association. 'We all just did what we were told,' Mrs Hall recalls. It was against the rules, according to Mrs Hall, for the committee to take an interest in any patient's difficulties. Mrs Conan knew everyone and, as a nurse herself, would have been able to advise the regularly changing nurses about things to watch out for. This empathy with the nurses would have been a great advantage within the association. Mrs Hall said the nurses were allocated different parts of the district, one taking Ballybrack and one in Dalkey. She remembers the new council house being organised by Dr Enright, the dispensary doctor. It was furnished by the committee with bits and pieces from everyone, and new beds were purchased. She said that modern nurses would not have been as pleased, but the two nurses were delighted not to be in 'digs'. The dispensary doctor was based in the Main Street in Dalkey village. The monthly meetings were held in people's homes, particularly in Mrs Fitzpatrick's house. Joan Hall also remembered meeting upstairs over the cake shop on Dalkey Road. The half day for shops and businesses in Dalkey was Wednesday, and they would meet then. The nurses came along to give a report when necessary. Mrs Purcell felt there was a little resentment of this by the nurses at the time.

She began in the district nursing association in 1960 and found that door-to-door collections were becoming increasingly difficult. Districts nearby had a public health nurse and did not have to pay, so it was hard to justify this voluntary provision in their area. Even though she was collecting in a very wealthy suburb of Dublin, she found that, towards the end of the scheme, there were more and more excuses for not contributing. Fundraising comprised the already-mentioned subscriptions and grants, and then the sale of work every year, featuring the usual cakes, jams and plant cuttings. The association also held an annual coffee evening in the Allied Irish Bank; the bank managers' wife, Mrs Minnis, was a supporter of the association. Our interviewees remember one nurse's dance in Killiney Castle and the time that Miss Atkins, Killiney opened her garden for a day. In November 1958 the *Irish Times* advertised a fashion show by 'The Mother and Baby Shop' to be held at the Cliff Castle Hotel, Dalkey in aid of the Jubilee nurses, for which tickets were priced at 3/-.[74] Mrs Hall said it was becoming increasingly clear that the association would not be able to afford the nurses' salaries and so it had to close in 1966.[75] It would have been closed down shortly thereafter in any event.

Fanad Health Club, County Donegal

Set up in 1932 for a population of 4,401 on the rural, very scenic Fanad peninsula in north Donegal, this association had two nurses, one in the upper part of the district and the other in the lower part. The president was Rev. Canon Gallagher, parish priest of Tamney. He died and was replaced by Rev. Alan Murray, Parochial House, Tamney. The treasurer was S.M. MacMenamin and the honourable secretaries were Miss E.R.C. Harte, Carrablagh and Mrs G. Barton, Dunfinny, Portsalon.

Miss Hart's papers, left with the Donegal Archives, show the extensive enquiries and effort required in the initial set-up of a district nursing association. Securing affiliation and a nurse from the Queen's Institute required much correspondence. Mrs Hart was relentless in her pursuit of grants and money-making schemes.

As a health club, the primary method of raising finance to sustain two nurses in a large, but not densely populated, rural area was through collections. An article at the time in the *Nursing Mirror and Midwives Journal* observed that it was essential to supplement collections with fundraisers.

> The countryside also turns out in force to support the honorary secretaries and founders, Miss Hart and Mrs G. Barton, when Miss Hart opens in aid of funds her beautiful grounds and still more beautiful walled garden.[76]

Nurses for this district began with Kathleen Clancy and Margaret O'Dowd, both newly qualified from St Laurence's Home and described by Miss Colburn of the Queen's Institute as two really good nurses. They arrived with their special nurse's bags and necessary books off the early mail train, reaching Letterkenny at 12.10.[77] Kathleen Clancy had to leave in 1937 because of ill health, at which point Mary Fitzgerald came from Carraroe, County Galway and remained until 1946. She left for other work and was replaced by Elizabeth Trainor, who stayed with the association until it closed in 1966. In 1946 Elizabeth Trainor became Mrs McGonigle. Margaret O'Dowd was transferred in 1935 and Mary Walshe stayed in Fanad until she was transferred to Limerick in 1938. Her replacement was Mary Guerin for three years and then Ann Cavanagh stayed for five years before her marriage. Bridget Conduff, who was newly qualified from St Laurence's Home and left in 1957 after seven years, was replaced by Margaret Trearty. Margaret married also and stayed in the district as Mrs Kerr until the association closed in 1966.

Inspections show that funds were low from about 1959. In 1964 the local authorities paid the committee's overdraft, and by November 1966 Miss Burke observed that the association had 'an overdraft and no means to pay the salaries yet'. It closed some weeks later.

Wicklow District Nursing Association

This association was affiliated in 1950 for a population of 6,000. Wicklow, now a large seaside town on the east coast of Ireland, was at the time a relatively small, insular community with a rural and coastal hinterland. The president of the association was Dr Aubrey O'Connor, The Ivies, Wicklow; Mrs Dawson, Bayview was the chairman; Mrs Shane of Churchill was secretary and Mrs O'Byrne, Ardmore was treasurer. The association provided a furnished house for the nurse in the town.

The first nurse, Mary Gorman, qualified in St Patrick's Home and stayed with the association until 1959 when she was transferred away. For a short while Therese O'Donnell stayed before taking a public health post. Finally, Mary Kiernan came from Newtownmountkennedy, County Wicklow in October 1959 and remained until the association closed in 1967. Mary Kiernan's story is celebrated in Chapter 1. Inspections of the district, noted as one short line in the Queen's Institute records, show a series of problems in Wicklow. There seem to have been snags from the very beginning. Miss Delaney noted that they had not received their grants yet in 1951. The committee members were disagreeing among themselves in 1954. A new committee was formed in 1955 and that year the nurse got her own car. In 1957, as with many committees, it was under pressure to accept midwifery work for the grant. In 1962 Telefís Éireann came to do a feature on the district and Miss Quain, Queen's Institute Superintendent for Ireland, made a special visit. The tape of the television interview with Nurse Kiernan, however, was sadly destroyed. Yet despite all of their troubles they survived until 1967 and Nurse Kiernan became the public health nurse for the area.

Donegal

There were a total of 40 district nursing associations throughout Donegal, each with their own nurse, working independently. For a short period they had a special support system similar to the county nursing associations that operated in England.[78]

Several nurses in Donegal were provided by the Lady Dudley's Scheme but many more were local voluntary associations and quite a few called themselves health clubs.

In September 1932 Dr Seán Ó Deagha, the first County Medical Officer in Donegal, set up an organisation that would help him, he hoped, to provide a voluntary nurse in every district in his area. He called it the Donegal County Nursing Association. He wrote to the secretary of all existing associations and health clubs asking for representatives to be appointed to this committee. The plan was to provide mutual support for both the committees of associations and the nurses themselves. The main objectives were to form new district nursing associations all over the county, to hold an annual reunion of nurses and to keep a fully stocked 'linen' cupboard so that each nurse could draw upon this when necessary. The Donegal County Nursing Association had two initial gatherings, one in Rosapenna in 1935 and one at Lough Eske in 1936. Nurses gathered from all over the county and good days were had by all, it seems. The first annual report of the association, year ending 1936, recorded the severe setback for the association on the death of Dr O'Dea (previously mentioned as Dr Seán Ó Deagha), 'so that as much progress as was anticipated has not been accomplished'.[79] Even the dance held in Ballybofey in November was not a great success. Flag days were held in very few districts.[80] Funding for local communities was, it appears, much easier than for an overall county body, no matter how logical it was. The association had the Countess of Mayo and Lord Bishop of Raphoe as their patrons and Miss Hart of Carrablagh, Portsalon was the president. Mrs Fullerton, Ramelton was the secretary, while vice-presidents included Lady Stewart of Ramelton and Mrs Boyd of Lifford. The other vice-presidents were Captain Hamilton of Ballintra, Mrs Dickson of Fahan and Mrs Bushe of Rathmullan.[81]

There was a very successful gathering held in Portsalon on 24 June 1937. The arrival of Miss Coburn, superintendent, and Miss Kavanagh, inspector, capped the day. Photographs were taken by the press and nurses looked spruce and lovely in their uniforms. Delegates from the associations also attended. The committee ladies wore their best coat and fur – if they had one – for the photograph, and hats and gloves were imperative. Miss Coburn addressed the meeting, hoping this would be an example to other counties to increase their numbers.

By July 1938 there was a little tension, however. A letter to the editor of the *Derry Journal* on 11 July 1938 by Captain J. Hamilton asked if it was necessary for the nurses to wear their uniform on the Bundoran outing. This was their holiday and they had expressed a wish not to have to wear their uniforms on the day. He said few delegates had turned up and the nurses had tried to enjoy themselves as best they could.[82]

The last of the documents left in the Donegal Archives in relation to this committee is a reference in the County Medical Officer's report of 1962. It says briefly: 'Apparently in pre-war days there was a federation of Voluntary Nursing Associations in County Donegal.'[83]

Donegal, because of the large number of nurses in the county, had a special representative on the council of the institute with responsibility for all of the Jubilee and Lady Dudley nurses, retired and otherwise. Mr Michael Chance of Newtowncunningham, County Donegal said in an interview that his earliest memories were of visiting elderly Jubilee nurses with his mother.[84] It was probably necessary to call regularly to nurses in isolated areas of Donegal, especially in the later stages of the scheme. Mr Chance said his mother was greeted with great affection and received Christmas cards every year from the nurses. His memory was of going to islands and seaside places on his summer holidays and recalls that it was a very positive experience. He also said that, even as a child, he observed that some of the nurses' home conditions were quite uncomfortable and that they relied greatly on the support of neighbours. Mrs Chance, along with her brother-in-law who lived in Dublin, became members of the Queen's Institute in the 1960s. The minutes of a Lady Dudley's committee meeting in July 1968 includes the following: 'Mrs Chance said she visited Arranmore Island and said Miss Smyth was a very good nurse. She had an interview with the Parish Priest who promised to have a collection in aid of our funds.'[85]

FORMER QUEEN'S NURSES

B.M. Hedderman

B.M. Hedderman was not qualified as a Queen's nurse in Ireland but her story was very similar to those of many Lady Dudley nurses at the time. She wrote a book, published in 1917, which outlined her experiences on the Aran Islands at the beginning of the twentieth century, entitled *Glimpses of My Life in Aran: Some Experiences of a District Nurse in those Remote Islands off the Coast of Ireland.*[86]

Nurse Hedderman does not illuminate any of her previous life except that she had been a district nurse in a 'large city'. She was not registered in the Roll of Jubilee Nurses so her history is unclear but she was probably appointed to the Aran Islands as midwife to one of the 723 dispensary districts set up after the establishment of the Poor Law Commission in 1852. Nurse Hedderman is noted in Mr William L. Micks' book, published in 1925, on the Congested Districts Board. She was appointed as one of three Irish-speaking teachers of domestic economy in the congested districts and was stationed at Achill Island.[87]

Annie Mary Patricia Smithson

Annie Mary Patricia Smithson was a Jubilee nurse from 1901 to 1920, having received training in both London and Edinburgh. Nurse Smithson had experience in many types of districts. Her first district service was as holiday relief in July and August 1901 in Portadown, County Down. She was then sent to Gilford, also in Down, for five years. Nurse Smithson was at this stage offered training in the Coombe Hospital in Dublin as a midwife, which was paid for by the Queen's Institute. Upon receiving her qualifications in midwifery, she was sent to Newmarket-on-Fergus, County Clare from 1907 to 1910. Glencolmcille, County Donegal was the only district in which she acted as a Lady Dudley's nurse where she spent eighteen months between 1910 and 1912. Nurse Smithson left that district without giving notice and was then appointed as a special tuberculosis nurse for the Women's National Health Association in Dublin from 1912 to 1913 before going to Clara, King's County (now Offaly) for one year. She then spent from May 1915 to April 1917 in Ballina, County Mayo and finally Dundrum, County Dublin from April 1917 to June 1919. It was recorded that she left for other work. In 1920 she re-joined the Queen's Institute and was sent to Waterford city.[88] She says she was supervised by a district nursing association committee but was paid directly by the corporation as a health visitor. Her next position was no longer under the auspices of the Queen's Institute. Invited by Dr

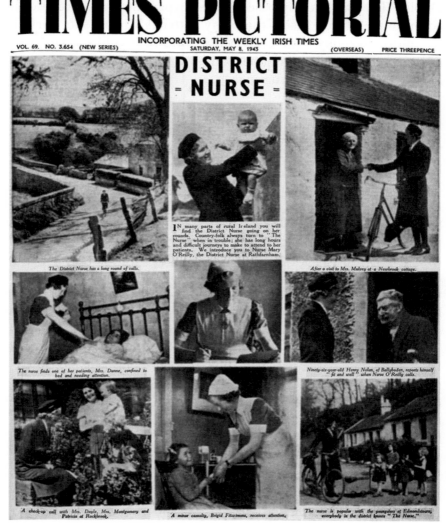

Courtesy of the *Irish Times*.

Alice Barry, she became the nurse for St Patrick's Baby Club which had been set up under the patronage of the Women's National Health Association. She was employed there for another eight years by Dublin Corporation as a childcare health worker. Nurse Smithson was very politically aware and became secretary of the Irish Nurses Organisation from 1929 to 1942. She wrote nineteen romantic and nationalist novels, all published by Talbot Press in Dublin. They are closely based on her experiences and provide an accurate picture of life in the many districts where she worked. Her autobiography, *Myself and Others*, was first published in 1944 after her death and is an honest and intimate representation of a Jubilee nurse in many situations.[89]

Emily Gillespie

The Roll of Jubilee Nurses describes Emily Gillespie's father as a bookseller. Educated in the Convent of Mercy, Strabane, County Tyrone and through private tuition, she trained as a general nurse in St Vincent's Hospital, Dublin from 1895 to 1900 and as a district nurse in St Laurence's Home in 1901. She was described on graduating as an 'energetic nurse who takes a great interest in her patients, conscientious and painstaking'. Mallow District Nursing Association in County Cork was her first district. She continued with them until retirement in 1922 for reasons of ill health. The honorary secretary of her committee, Isadora Webb, came to Dublin and put a note in her records on the roll upon Emily's retirement. 'It is a cause of great concern to the members of the committee, to the doctors and patients that she now finds it impossible, for health reasons, to continue her work.'[90] Nurse Gillespie was indeed well regarded in her community, as described by Mrs William O'Brien in her memoirs in 1937. 'The Jubilee nurse had a sturdy spirit of her northern race, if it was tempered with a delightful touch of gentleness. She worked on in Mallow until she became part of it. She found her way to every heart.'[91]

Mary Quain

Mary Quain was born in Galbally, County Limerick in 1911. She trained as a general nurse in the South Charitable Infirmary and County Hospital in Cork city. She went from there to the Rotunda Hospital in Dublin to train as a midwife and across the road in Parnell Square to St Laurence's Home where she graduated as a Queen's nurse in April 1937. Superintendent Colburn described her as a 'conscientious kindly nurse, very gentle and considerate with the patients'.[92] It was noted that Nurse Quain had the Irish language and was a cyclist. Her first two assignments involved temporary summer relief in Bealadangan and Lettermullen, both in County Galway, in 1937. In the autumn of that year she started as a permanent Lady Dudley's nurse in Carraroe, County Galway. Carraroe was one of the busiest midwifery districts in the country at the time. After six years, Nurse Quain was transferred to Keel in Achill Island, County Mayo where she remained for a further five years. Her next district was her first experience working with a district nursing committee, at Glengarriff in west Cork.[93] It was originally financed by Lady Dudley's Scheme but in 1927 a district nursing committee was set up under the presidency of Mrs Leigh-White of Bantry House.[94] Nurse Quain was transferred to Youghal in east Cork after one year in west Cork and she remained there for two years. She received a silver badge in 1951 from the Queen's Institute. She was promoted to acting superintendent at St Patrick's Home for District Nursing and on completion of a course in special administrative expertise in Edinburgh she was advanced to superintendent of the home.[95] In 1959 Miss Quain became the last superintendent of the Queen's Institute of Ireland and she retired to Rathfarnham, Dublin until her death in 1999.

Mary Agnes O'Grady

Mary Agnes O'Grady was from Ballaghaderreen, County Roscommon. Born in 1903, her father, like that of many Jubilee nurses, was a farmer. She attended secondary school in the Mercy Convent, Baggot Street, Dublin and trained in general nursing at Sir Patrick Dunn's Hospital, Dublin between 1926 and 1929. She worked as a staff nurse there and in Birmingham before training to be a midwife in the Rotunda Hospital, Dublin. St Patrick's Home in St Stephen's Green was where she completed her path to becoming a Queen's nurse in 1936. Miss Colburn, the superintendent for St Patrick's Home, wrote in her graduation report: 'Miss O Grady is a thoroughly well-trained nurse. Most kindly and considerate with patients by whom she is much respected and truly liked. The nurse is capable of teaching her patients and their friends as she has grasped the wider responsibilities of our work.'[96] Nurse O'Grady's first district was her last. She began to nurse in Ballinasloe, County Galway shortly after finishing her training and continued to care for the people of the town and its hinterland until her death in 1955.

Phyllis Nelson (nee Sproule)

Phyllis Nelson was originally from Sligo but trained as a general nurse at the Adelaide Hospital in Dublin. She worked as a staff nurse in St Patrick's in Sligo before training in psychiatric nursing in St Brendan's Hospital at Grangegorman in Dublin. She went to London to train as a midwife in the Mother's Hospital in Clapton. Phyllis trained as a Jubilee nurse in St Patrick's Nurses' Home in 1963 and worked as a staff nurse and deputy superintendent at the home upon its relocation to Morehampton Road, Donnybrook, Dublin until she 'left for marriage' in 1967.[97]

Mary Catherine Byrne (nee McGuinness)

From Coolaney, County Sligo, Mary Byrne trained as a general nurse in St Laurence's Hospital in Dublin. She did her midwifery training in the Coombe Maternity Hospital also in Dublin and trained as a Jubilee nurse in St Patrick's Nurses' Home at Morehampton Road. Mary's first district was Naas, County Kildare for one year. Both Queen's Institute inspections described her as 'well trained, cheerful, conscientious and popular with patients'.[98] She subsequently completed a public health course and moved to Mayo to work as a public health nurse.

Jenny Ledingham

Jenny Ledingham began life in Mornington, County Louth. She trained in the Royal Victoria Hospital in Belfast and staffed there for a short period before moving to the Jubilee and City Hospital, Belfast for her maternity training. Nurse Ledingham trained as a Jubilee nurse in St Patrick's Nurses Home in 1964. Until 1967, when the home closed, she was based in St Patrick's as a supervising district nurse in the Crumlin Dispensary, Cashel Road, Dublin.[99] She then worked as a hospital nurse in England for a few years and returned to Dublin to do the public health course in St Stephen's Green. This was a nine-month course run by Miss Morgan, the last superintendent of St Patrick's Nurses' Home and was run by An Bord Altranais. Employed by the Department of Health, she worked at Kilbarrack in Dublin. She now lives in Pembroke in Wales.[100]

Jenny was inspired by her aunt, Annie Law Ledingham, who was also a Jubilee nurse in Enniskillen, County Fermanagh. Annie received her Longstanding Badge in 1966 having served in her district for 21 years.

Ann Mary Connolly (nee Barry)

Ann Barry was originally from Limerick and did her general nursing there at the Regional Hospital, Dooradoyle. She went back as a staff nurse for a short while after qualifying as a midwife at the Rotunda Lying-in Hospital, Dublin. After qualifying as a Queen's nurse at St Patrick's Nurses' Home she was sent to the district nursing association at Kilmeaden, County Waterford.[101] Upon closure of the district in 1967, Nurse Barry completed the two-month public health course in order to continue as a district nurse, employed by the local county council.

Bridget Bernadette Hartery (nee Coleman)

Bridget Hartery, from Mullinavat, County Kilkenny, trained as a general nurse at Ardkeen Hospital in Waterford and qualified as a midwife at the National Maternity Hospital, Holles Street, Dublin. Bridget worked as a staff nurse for a short period in Jersey and St Patrick's Hospital, Waterford before training as a Jubilee nurse. After she qualified in St Patrick's Home she was sent temporarily to Greystones District Nursing Association in County Wicklow. The Greystones committee would have liked to keep Nurse Coleman but she was sent to Tramore, County Waterford as a permanent post.[102] It turned out to be not that permanent as, like the others, her district was closed down, but her work continued seamlessly as a public health nurse in the same area. She continued to be involved in public health services in the Waterford area until her retirement.

Bridget Philomena Fennelly (nee Meally)

From Castlecomer, County Kilkenny, Bridget Fennelly went to Ardkeen Hospital in Waterford to train as a general nurse. Her training in midwifery was completed in Stobhill in Glasgow and she stayed on as a staff nurse in the British Nursing Association for a short period. Nurse Meally then went to St Patrick's Home to train as a Queen's nurse. She was kept as a temporary staff nurse with them before being transferred to her district in Cashel, County Tipperary. Once again, despite having a popular and pleasant nurse,[103] Cashel District Nursing Association closed in 1970 on the marriage of Nurse Meally.

Mary Rita Kiernan

Born in Dunleer, County Louth in 1912, Mary Kiernan was the daughter of a farmer. Her mother died young and Mary was sent to boarding school at Mount Anville, Dublin. She completed her general nursing in St Vincent's Hospital, Dublin and trained as a midwife in the National Maternity Hospital, Holles Street, Dublin. She was a staff nurse there before beginning her district training in St Patrick's Home to qualify as a Queen's nurse in July 1937. It was noted in her final assessment by the superintendent Miss Colburn that her ambition since childhood had been to become a Jubilee nurse. She began at St Anne's District Nursing Association in Inniscarra, County Cork from 1937 until 1939 when she was transferred to the less rural district of Cahir, County Tipperary for another three years. Mary took a break at this stage, handing in her badge, to work in a hospital post. She re-joined the Queen's Institute after less than a year to be placed with Dunboyne District Nursing Association, County Meath. She was keen and well liked by the people and her committee but had to leave because of 'home duties' within the same year. Once again, Mary returned to the Queen's Institute to reclaim her badge and begin on a district in

1949. Newtownmountkennedy and the surrounding townlands in County Wicklow were the lucky recipients of Nurse Kiernan's doubtless energies. She remained for ten years on that district until 1959 and was then transferred to the nearby town of Wicklow. She continued as Jubilee nurse in Wicklow town and its countryside for another ten years until the district closed in 1967, at which point she became their public health nurse.[104] A bench outside the cottage hospital commemorated, on behalf of the grateful people of Wicklow, the long contribution of Mary Kiernan to the town. It was, however, subsequently stolen.

Maura Kilmartin (nee McLoughlin)

Maura Kilmartin was born in Red Barns, Dundalk in County Louth. She was educated in the Ursuline Convent, Sligo and trained as a general nurse in the Meath Hospital, Dublin and as a midwife in the National Maternity Hospital, Holles Street, Dublin. She worked as a midwife in Holles Street Hospital for another year before training as a district nurse. She qualified as a Jubilee nurse from St Laurence's Home in 1952. In her report when Maura McLoughlin completed her training, Miss Aylward the superintendent said that she 'presents a good professional manner'.[105] Nurse McLoughlin was given a choice of first district, either Castlecomer, County Waterford – where she had been doing holiday relief – or Dundrum, County Dublin. She chose Dundrum because it was easier for her mother, who had been recently widowed, to visit on public transport. It was, at the time, a village outside Dublin city with a very rapidly growing population. She married the vice-principal of the local national school and continued on the district despite her married status. She took leave of absence when her daughter was born and was asked by the committee to return when her daughter was four years old. In 1968 when the district nursing association was given notice to end activities, Mrs Kilmartin had to attend an interview for a public health post in the area. At the time she had concerns, despite her great experience, as no other married nurse was going for the interview. She continued, however, to work as a public health nurse in Dundrum district until her retirement.

Mary Catherine Duffy (nee Kearns)

Mary Duffy was born in a farm called Carronmorris, Dromard in County Sligo. She went to a local school and came to Dublin to train as a nurse. Following in the footsteps of her aunt Linda Kearns McWinney, she trained in Dr Stephens's Hospital from 1938. The National Maternity Hospital was where she trained as a midwife until 1944. Her aunt had set up a private nursing cooperative in Gardiner Place in Dublin and she worked with them for some time. Following a temporary public health posting in Lord Edward Street, Dublin, Mary Kearns decided to train as a Jubilee nurse. Miss Colburn said in her final report: 'Miss Kearns is a capable, well-trained, energetic nurse. Obviously trusted and very much liked by the patients and their friends. Nurse possesses a particularly good professional manner. Her ready smile and kindly sympathetic ways endear her to all.'[106] In 1945 she was sent to Taughboyne district in Donegal and, according to the records, she left for marriage in 1951. Mary Duffy said in her memoirs that she occasionally covered annual leave or sick leave for the nurses in the area when her children were young. Having moved to

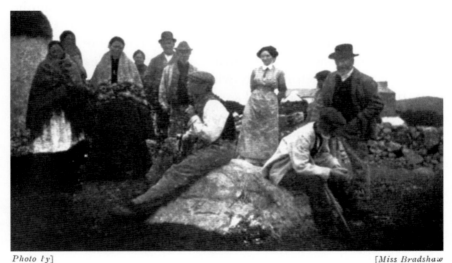

Photo ly]   [*Miss Bradshaw*

DISPENSARY DAY, CARNA.
Courtesy of National Library of Ireland.

Newtowncunningham with her family, the district nursing association of that district asked her to return to work in 1965 and she did so in January 1966. The committee decided not to close with the Queen's Institute in 1967 and remained open until 1974. Mrs Duffy then applied to be a public health nurse until she retired.

Rita Anne Pearson (nee McAuley)

Rita Pearson, originally from Drumbeg in County Donegal, began her general nurse training in 1942 in the City Hospital, Belfast. She also trained as a midwife in Belfast and worked as a staff nurse there for a further year. Following this, she claims to have developed 'itchy feet' and travelled to London where she staffed in the London Chest Hospital as a tuberculosis nurse. She trained as a Queen's nurse in Rochdale, Lancashire and worked on the district for two years. She worked as a Jubilee nurse in Randalstown, County Antrim for two years between 1949 and 1952 before her marriage to a Donegal farmer. Randalstown was one of the last districts to be affiliated in the North of Ireland but was taken over by the National Health Scheme for Northern Ireland in 1948.[107] The policy at the time was to let the district nursing association committee continue its work but with no financial obligations to fund the nurse. Following a career break, she continued to work as a night sister in Altnagelvin Hospital in Derry in the early 1960s. Rita Pearson lived in Johnstown which was part of the district of Taughboyne, Carrigens.[108] When the district lost its Jubilee nurse in 1961, Nurse Pearson offered to stay for a short time. She continued in that district until the committee closed and then as public health nurse for a total of sixteen years. Later she set up a private nursing home in Holywood, County Down but is now enjoying her retirement.[109]

The following photographs were taken by Mr Conrad Pim, committee member of Lady Dudley's Scheme, who travelled around Ireland recording the nurses at their 'station' in 1935.

This collection of photographs is held at the National Archives of Ireland.

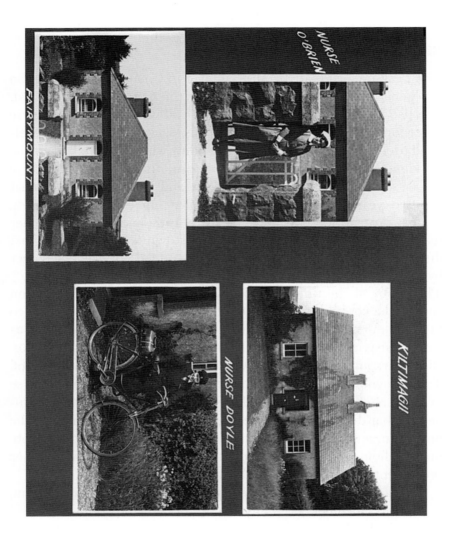

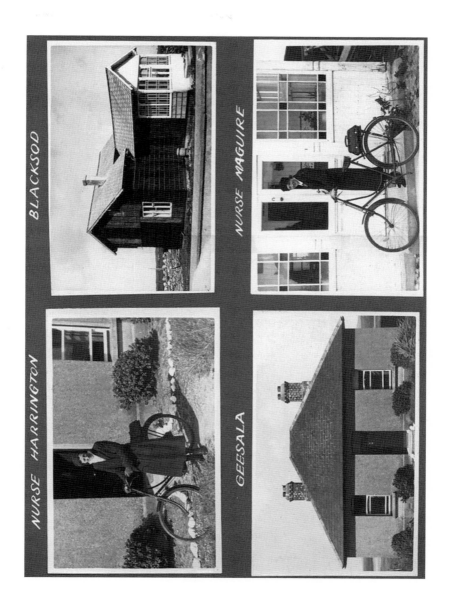

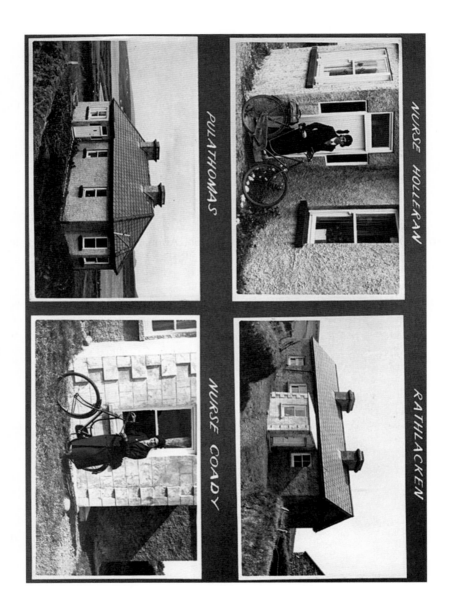

NOTES

1   Airfield Archives are now in the care of Maynooth Archive and Research Centre, Castletown House, Celbridge, Co. Kildare. OPW/NUI, Reference Number PP/AIR.

2   Jubilee Nurses, Affiliated Branches, P220/28, pp. 289–90. An Bord Altranais Archives, UCD.

3   Dundrum District Nursing Association, Annual Report, 1961. Airfield Archives, OPW/NUI, PP/AIR.

4   Jubilee Nurses, Affiliated Branches, P220/29, pp. 427–9. An Bord Altranais Archives, UCD.

5   Dundrum District Nursing Association, Annual Reports. Airfield Archives, OPW/NUI, PP/AIR.

6   Ibid., ledgers.

7   Ibid., annual reports.

8   Ibid.

9   Jubilee Nurses, Affiliated Branches, P220/29, pp. 427–9. An Bord Altranais Archives, UCD.

10   Dundrum District Nursing Association, Annual Report, 1921. Airfield Archives, OPW/NUI, PP/AIR.

11   Dundrum District Nursing Association, Airfield Archives, OPW/NUI, PP/AIR.

12   Roll of Jubilee Nurses, P220/31, vol. 1, p. 47. An Bord Altranais Archives, UCD.

13   Annie P. Smithson, *Myself and Others* (Dublin: The Talbot Press, 1945), p. 235.

14   *Queen's Nurses' Magazine* (April 1918), The Queen's Nursing Institute, London.

15   Smithson, *Myself and Others*, p. 239.

16   Ibid., p. 241.

17   Roll of Jubilee Nurses, P220/31, vol. 1, p. 63. An Bord Altranais Archives, UCD.

18   Ibid., p. 168.

19   Jubilee Nurses, Affiliated Branches, P220/29, pp. 427–9. An Bord Altranais Archives, UCD.

20   Department of Health files A10/50 and M104/113. National Archives, Dublin.

21   Annual Reports of Dundrum District Nursing Association, Airfield Archives, OPW/NUI, PP/AIR.

22   Roll of Jubilee Nurses, P220/36, vol. 6, p. 192. An Bord Altranais Archives, UCD.

23   Jubilee Nurses, Affiliated Branches, P220–9, pp. 427–9. An Bord Altranais Archives, UCD.

24   Interviews with Maura Kilmartin, July, August and October 2011.

25 Dundrum District Nursing Association. Airfield Archives, OPW/NUI, PP/AIR.

26 Dundrum District Nursing Association, Annual Report, 1967. A copy of this, and the 1966 report, are now in the possession of the author, with gratitude to Mrs Kilmartin.

27 This hall had been recently built with a donation from Letitia Overend for St John Ambulance Brigade.

28 Dundrum District Nursing Association. Airfield Archives, OPW/NUI, PP/AIR.

29 Ibid.

30 *Irish Times*, 11 December 1895, p. 6. Irish Times Archives.

31 Elizabeth, Countess of Fingall, *Seventy Years Young* (Dublin: The Lilliput Press, 1991).

32 Annual Report for Fr Healy DNA, Bray, 1950. Department of Health files, M100/132. National Archives, Dublin.

33 Roll of Jubilee Nurses, P220/29, vol. 1, p. 123. An Bord Altranais Archives, UCD.

34 Mrs William O'Brien, *My Irish Friends* (Dublin and London: Burns Oates & Washbourne, 1937), p. 115. Sophie O'Brien, nee Raffalovich (1860–1960), was born in Odessa, Russia to a wealthy Jewish family. Her family moved to Paris in 1863, so her formative years were spent in France. She married William O'Brien (1852–1928) in 1890. Originally from Mallow, Co. Cork, he had been editor of the Irish Land League newspaper *United Ireland*, and was a member of the British parliament before the formation of the Irish Free State. Mrs O'Brien went back to France a few years after the death of her husband, where she lived in relative poverty until her death. Cork City Archives.

35 Ibid.

36 Ibid., p. 117.

37 Ibid., p. 120.

38 Interview with Mr Rory Kilduff, Ballinasloe, Co. Galway, 6 August 2010.

39 Ibid.

40 Department of Health files, M104/8. National Archives, Dublin

41 Interview with Mr Mathew Ganly, Ballinasloe, Co. Galway, 6 August 2010

42 Ibid.

43 *The Kildare Observer*, 20 October 1928, p. 9. News Plan Database, National Library, Dublin.

44 Ibid., 13 February 1931, p. 6.

45 Ibid., 9 April 1927, p. 5.

46 Ibid., 18 July 1930, p. 6.

47 Ibid., 23 February 1929, p. 5.

48 Annual Report for Portmarnock, Baldoyle DNA, 1949. Department of Health files, M100/132. National Archives, Dublin.

49   Birr Castle Archives, Letter 9 February 1947. These documents are in the safekeeping of Lord and Lady Rosse of Birr Castle. This is a private collection and it is not generally available.

50   Ibid.

51   *Queen's Nurses' Magazine* (August 1908), p. 93. The Queen's Nursing Institute, London.

52   Birr Castle Archives, handwritten minute book, 13 September 1945.

53   Jubilee Nurses, Affiliated Branches, P220/28, vol. 1, pp. 559–62. An Bord Altranais Archives, UCD.

54   Roll of Jubilee Nurses, P220/36, vol. 6, p. 101. An Bord Altranais Archives, UCD.

55   Obituary of Mrs Doolan by Anne the Countess of Rosse. Received by the author from Mr Joseph H. McGrath, son-in-law of Mrs Doolan.

56   Birr Castle Archives, handwritten letter, 27 November 1967, to Nurse McEvoy from Dr A. Reeves, County Medical Officer.

57   Birr Castle Archives.

58   Jubilee Nurses, Affiliated Branches, P220/30, vol. 3, pp. 301–2. An Bord Altranais Archives, UCD.

59   Box P48/1–3.Donegal Archives, Lifford, Co. Donegal.

60   Minute books, 1945–74, Box P48/1–3. Donegal Archives, Lifford, Co. Donegal.

61   Telephone interview with Mr Michael Chance, 18 January 2012.

62   Group interview in the home of Mr and Mrs Chance, Manorcunningham, Co. Donegal, 11 August 2011.

63   Jubilee Nurses, Affiliated Branches, P220/30, vol. 3, pp. 301–2. An Bord Altranais Archives, UCD.

64   Newtowncunningham, Burt, Killea DNA, Annual Report, 29 February 1952, Box P48/1–3. Donegal Archives, Lifford, Co. Donegal.

65   Group interview in the home of Mr and Mrs Chance, Manorcunningham, County Donegal, 11 August 2011.

66   Minute books, 1945–74, Box P48/1–3. Donegal Archives, Lifford, Co. Donegal.

67   Interview in the home of Michael and Kate Chance, Manorcunningham, Co. Donegal, 11 August 2011.

68   Minute books, 1945–74, Box P48/1–3. Donegal Archives, Lifford, Co. Donegal.

69   Group interview in the home of Mr and Mrs Chance, Manorcunningham, County Donegal, 11 August 2011.

70   Minute books, 1945–74, Box P48/1–3. Donegal Archives, Lifford, Co. Donegal.

71   Group interview in the home of Mr and Mrs Chance, Manorcunningham, County Donegal, 11 August 2011.

72   Newtowncunningham, Burt, Killea DNA, Annual Report, May 1968, Box P48/1–3. Donegal Archives, Lifford, Co. Donegal.

73   Telephone interview with Mrs Rita Pearson, 27 October 2011.

74   *Irish Times*, 1 November 1958, p. 14. Irish Times Archives.

75   Interview with Mrs Joan Hall and Mrs Anne Purcell, 20 July 2011.

76   'In Wildest Donegal', p. 28.

77   Correspondence between Miss Hart, Portsalon, Co. Donegal and QIDNI, Dublin, 23 May 1932, Box P27/10. Donegal Archives, Lifford, Co. Donegal.

78   Howse, 'The Ultimate Destination of All Nursing'.

79   First Annual Report and accounts of the Donegal County Nursing Association, 1936. Miss Harte documents, Box P27/10. Donegal Archives, Lifford, Co. Donegal.

80   Ibid.

81   Ibid.

82   All documents in relation to this committee were found in Box P27/10. Donegal Archives, Lifford, Co. Donegal.

83   Annual Report, County Medical Officer, Donegal, 1962/3, p. 86. Donegal Archives, Lifford, Co. Donegal.

84   Group interview in the home of Mr and Mrs Chance, Manorcunningham, Co. Donegal, 11 August 2011.

85   Lady Dudley's Committee, Minutes of Monthly Meetings, July 1968, M104/100. National Archives Dublin.

86   Hedderman, *Glimpses of My Life in Arran*.

87   Micks, *The Congested Districts Board for Ireland 1891–1923*, p. 94.

88   Roll of Jubilee Nurses, vol. 1, P220/31, p. 29. An Bord Altranais Archives, UCD.

89   Smithson, *Myself and Others*.

90   Roll of Jubilee Nurses, vol. 1, P220/31, p. 26. An Bord Altranais Archives, UCD.

91   O'Brien, *My Irish Friends*, pp. 115–16.

92   Roll of Jubilee Nurses, vol. 4, P220/34, p. 142. Bord Altranais Archives, UCD.

93   Ibid.

94   Jubilee Nurses, Affiliated Branches, P220/27, pp. 511–14. An Bord Altranais Archives, UCD.

95   Roll of Jubilee Nurses, vol. 4, P220/34, p. 142. An Bord Altranais Archives, UCD.

96   Ibid., p. 109.

97   Roll of Jubilee Nurses, vol. 4, P220/37, p. 109. An Bord Altranais Archives, UCD.

98   Ibid., p. 151.

99   Roll of Jubilee Nurses, vol. 7, P220/37, p. 136. An Bord Altranais Archives, UCD.

100   Interview with Jenny Ledingham, 13 August 2010.

101 Roll of Jubilee Nurses, vol. 7, P220/37, p. 158. An Bord Altranais Archives, UCD.

102 Ibid., p. 165.

103 Ibid., p.163.

104 Roll of Jubilee Nurses, vol. 4, P220/34, p. 143. An Bord Altranais Archives, UCD.

105 Roll of Jubilee Nurses, vol. 6, P220/36, p. 210. An Bord Altranais Archives, UCD.

106 Ibid., p. 93.

107 Queen's Institute of District Nursing, Northern Ireland Executive Committee, Annual Report, 1947, p. 5. QVJIN National Archives, Dublin.

108 Roll of Jubilee Nurses, vol. 7, P220/37, p. 181. An Bord Altranais Archives, UCD.

109 Telephone interview with Mrs Rita Pearson, 27 October 2011.

CHAPTER 5

Viceregal Patronage – Lady Dudley and Lady Aberdeen

LADY DUDLEY'S NURSING SCHEME FOR THE ESTABLISHMENT OF
DISTRICT NURSES IN THE POOREST PARTS OF IRELAND

Vice Regal Lodge

April 23rd 1903

Sir,

During the months I have spent in Ireland constant appeals have been made to me from the poorest and most congested parts of the country, for help towards providing District Nurses, and the great need for assisting the people in this direction has been brought home to me very forcibly in many different ways.

Queen Victoria's Jubilee Institute for Nurses provides for the thorough training of suitable District Nurses, and much excellent work is being done under its supervision in many places in Ireland, but it is obliged, except in a few special cases, to leave the maintenance of Nurses, once started, to local effort.

The average annual cost of maintenance of each Nurse is about £100, and it is just in those places where the need for such Nurses is greatest on account of the extreme poverty of the people that it is impossible to obtain the necessary funds locally. In many of the very poor districts there are no resident gentry and no well-to-do inhabitants of the middle classes, and because of their poverty the people themselves are not able to make any contribution.

I recently approached the Central Authority of Queen Victoria's Jubilee Institute for Nurses with a view to securing their cooperation in providing and maintaining Nurses in these districts, where the need for them is so acute, and I am happy to be able to announce that the Committee have generously voted a sum of £180 per annum to form the nucleus of a special fund to be raised for the purpose, and they have also undertaken to supervise the Nurses through their Dublin Branch.

Four Nurses, maintained by funds raised outside the neighbourhoods in which they work are already established in congested districts. Two are supported by a Manchester Fund, The West of Ireland Association, one by the Irish Homestead newspaper, and one in Achill mainly by Queen Victoria's Jubilee Institute. The work done by these Nurses is admirable, and my knowledge of the usefulness of their ministrations encourages me to appeal to the public for funds to provide similar assistance throughout the many other congested areas in Ireland.

I feel sure that all who know anything of the misery which prevails among the people in some of the poverty-stricken country districts, will recognise how much may be done for the relief of their immediate necessities, and the improvement of the conditions under which they live, by the establishment among them of thoroughly trained and capable District Nurses.

It is with confidence, therefore that I appeal for subscriptions to a fund to be expended in establishing and assisting to maintain Nurses in the poorest of the country districts of Ireland.

I shall be happy to receive contributions, in the form of Donations of Annual Subscriptions, or they may be sent to the Secretary of the Bank of Ireland, marked Lady Dudley's Fund for Jubilee Nurses.

Yours faithfully,

Rachel Dudley[1]

The Lady Dudley's Nursing Scheme for the Establishment of District Nurses in the Poorest Parts of Ireland (1903–74) was introduced by Lady Rachel Dudley, wife of William Ward, second Earl of Dudley and viceroy to Ireland from August 1902 until December 1905. It was a short term of office for the Dudleys in Ireland but one from which the poorest districts on the western seaboard were to benefit enormously. At this time, district nursing was becoming a widespread feature throughout the United Kingdom. In Dublin, the Irish branch of the Queen's Institute was established with two training homes – St Patrick's Protestant Training Home at 101 St

Stephen's Green and St Laurence's Catholic Training Home at 34 Rutland Square (now Parnell Square).

As part of their duty as Lord and Lady Lieutenant, the Earl and Countess of Dudley toured the country extensively. Lady Dudley was struck by the sheer plight and destitution of the agricultural poor in the rural districts on the western seaboard. Aware of the work of the Queen's Institute, she felt these people would benefit from the services of the Jubilee nurses. Under the guidelines of the Queen's Institute and its rules regarding the affiliation of associations, it was necessary for the community applying for a district nursing association to have the means of making contributions to the association in order for it to provide a nurse. The people of these communities had no such means and so Lady Dudley devised a plan to set up her own scheme – Lady Dudley's Scheme for the Establishment of District Nurses in the Poorest Parts of Ireland ("Lady Dudley's Scheme").

THE WEST OF IRELAND ASSOCIATION

Before Lady Dudley's visit to Ireland, a group of ladies based in Manchester had already taken an interest in the poverty-stricken districts of the west of Ireland, as representatives of the West of Ireland Association. This association was formed as an endeavour to bring industries to this area of Ireland and its objective was 'to stimulate in England an interest in the social and material wellbeing of the people in the congested districts of the West of Ireland, and to aim at the amelioration of their condition and the encouragement of self help'. When some members of its committee visited Ireland in the 1890s, they were appalled by the poverty facing the population in the west and sought to form the basis for some form of permanent nursing scheme.

In 1897, the year of Queen Victoria's diamond jubilee, the people of Manchester raised over £20,000. Using this money, the association appointed two Jubilee nurses under the control and supervision of the Queen's Institute, Nurse Josephine Bird to Oughterard, County Galway and Nurse Annie Henry to Burriscarra, County Mayo, both in 1899.[2] The Lady Dudley's Scheme took over the financial supervision of these nurses and their districts upon its establishment.

Foundation of the Scheme

By 1902, when Lady Dudley arrived in Ireland, the Queen's Institute was going from strength to strength with requests received from all over the country for district nurses. When the Earl of Dudley became lord lieutenant and viceroy to Ireland, his wife Lady Rachel Dudley was to follow in the footsteps of her two predecessors, Lady Ishbel Aberdeen and Lady Beatrix Cadogan, both of whom had been actively interested in the development of district nursing. Lady Cadogan was on the council of the Queen's Institute and Lady Aberdeen had helped to establish the Victorian Order of Nurses in Canada in 1897. The Dudleys were young and dynamic and already had a family of four children – two sons and two daughters – upon their arrival in Ireland. These were Gladys Honor (b. 1892), William Eric (b. 1894), Morvyth Lillian (b. 1896); and Roderick John (b. 1902). Three more children were later born

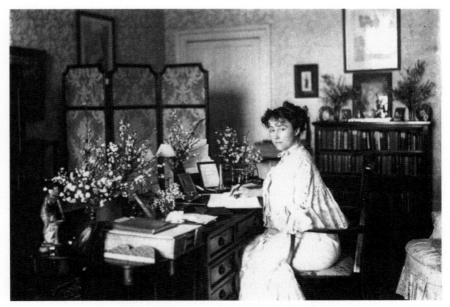

Courtesy of the Library Council of NSW, Australia.
Mitchell, State Library of NSW – ON 5/60.

– Alexandra Patricia (b. 1904) and twins Edward Frederick and George Reginald (b. 1907). Lady Rachel Dudley was described by Ada Holman, wife of the premier of New South Wales as 'beautiful as a marble statue … a carved lily'.[3]

LADY RACHEL DUDLEY

Early Life

Lady Rachel Dudley (1867–1920) was the daughter of Charles Henry Gurney of the Gurney banking family and Alice Gurney (nee Princep). She had a sister, Laura, who married and became Lady Troubridge and a brother, Henry Edward. Rachel's mother and father separated when she was very young. Later, in her obituary, the newspapers unkindly referred to her as 'the Shopgirl Countess', as she and her mother had established a millinery business in London which had failed.[4] Through her mother's connections she went to live with Lord and Lady Bedford, friends of Lady Aberdeen, during her late teens. It was while staying with the Bedfords that Rachel met the dashing William Humble Ward, the second Earl of Dudley, who was reputed to be a man of considerable wealth and connection. The young couple married in 1891 and their wedding was a society affair with the Prince of Wales, later to become Edward VII, in attendance.[5]

Lord and Lady Lieutenant for Ireland 1902–1995

Upon her death, Queen Victoria was succeeded by her son Edward VII and his wife Queen Alexandra, with whom the Dudleys maintained a friendship. When the Earl of Dudley was appointed lord lieutenant, the Earl and Lady Dudley travelled widely throughout Ireland and involved themselves in many Irish affairs as part of their duty as representatives of the King. They had a hunting villa, Screebe Lodge in Rosmuck, County Galway, which they often visited. It was during her travels throughout Ireland that Lady Dudley observed the poverty and destitution in which the poorer classes lived in the remote parts of the country and particularly in the congested districts in the west. The stone and mud cabins that the agricultural class lived in on the western seaboard were dire as dwellings. Photographs taken during this time speak for themselves. The people lived in hovels in dirt and squalor; they wore hardly any clothes, if any at all; they had no shoes and were often many miles away from their nearest neighbours. Infant mortality, disease and infection were the norm.

Accordingly, Lady Dudley set upon herself the task of endeavouring to introduce an organised system of trained district nurses to these places. She realised that these areas could neither afford to employ a nurse nor could any district nursing associations possibly be formed by the scattered inhabitants, and as she said in her letter above, 'there are no resident gentry and no well-to-do inhabitants of the middle classes' who could raise the necessary funding.

Lady Dudley, greatly moved by the appeals for help on behalf of the poor, decided to found an organisation to specifically address the problem. She was determined that the project would be established on a sound financial footing. She insisted that 'no nurse be appointed until the money necessary for her equipment is in the hands of the Committee and the yearly sum required for her maintenance guaranteed'.[6] In April 1903 Lady Dudley's Scheme for the Establishment of Districts in the Poorest Part of Ireland officially commenced.

First Committee of Lady Dudley's Nursing Scheme

Using her influential position as vicerine, Lady Dudley was able to put together a formidable committee, of which she herself was chairperson, which she could depend on to muster subscriptions and donations. This first committee consisted of a veritable mix of society, business, church and government personalities with royal interest an added benefit. The list of committee members was made up of the elite of local society, some of whom were also actively involved on the committees of St Patrick's Nurses Home, St Laurence's Nurses Home and the council of the Queen's Institute and were absolutely committed to enhancing the positive influence the Jubilee nurses were having on the wellbeing of the sick poor. Under this committee, Lady Dudley's Scheme was established with the assistance of subscriptions and donations from a network of benefactors and friends numbering nearly 500 people. Queen Alexandra, on an official visit to Ireland in August 1903, expressed interest in the plan and before leaving sent a donation to Lady Dudley with a note asking to be kept informed on the progress of the scheme.[7]

THE EARLY DAYS OF LADY DUDLEY'S SCHEME

17 August 1903 was a red letter day for the supporters of Lady Dudley's Scheme as it saw the deployment of its first two nurses – Nurse McCoy and Nurse Elizabeth Cusack at Geesala, County Mayo and Bealadangan, County Galway respectively. Geesala, in the parish of Bangor, aimed to serve a population of 2,000 scattered along a peninsula surrounded by a wide and desolate bog. Bealadangan, situated on a headland, connected many small islands with a densely populated area of around 3,500 and was one of the poorest districts in the country. Most of the inhabitants lived with their families in one-room residences in the form of stone hovels.[8]

The initial response to the appeal for funding of Lady Dudley's Scheme was considerable, and in the first year these initial two nurses were joined by a further seven, deployed throughout the west of Ireland.[9] Since 1897 Achill Island had been serviced by a Jubilee nurse. The island was the 39th district affiliated with the Queen's Institute and had been maintained by means of a special fund raised and administered by the institute. At the request of the institute in 1903 Lady Dudley's Scheme took over control of this district. Achill Island was highly populated, with a huge number of one-room cabins. The first report of Lady Dudley's Scheme listed them as follows: 32 occupied by 1 person; 59 by 2 persons; 42 by 3 persons; 40 by 4 persons; 19 by 5 persons; 23 by 6 persons; 15 by 7 persons; 6 by 8 persons; 2 by 9 persons; and 1 by 10 persons.[10]

The cost of keeping a nurse in the more remote agricultural districts, if a furnished cottage was to be provided, was £108 to £112 per annum which included rent and taxes, salary, uniform allowance, board, wages and allowance for the keep of a servant, fire and lighting. Initial sundry items such as bicycle or medical stores were a further £55. This cost was considerably smaller in districts where furnished lodgings were readily available. In some districts it was too rough for the use of a bicycle so the nurse was to be provided with a pony and cart. The nurses were also provided with comforts for very needy patients by way of a small store of Bovril, Liebig's Extract and Condensed Milk as fresh milk was often unobtainable.[11]

PUBLIC RELATIONS

The success of the first year gave the committee great encouragement and Lady Dudley personally began a public relations campaign in earnest. By 12 December 1903 she was writing again to the editor of *The Times* in appeal for some English Christmas charity.[12] She also wrote to the *New York Times* appealing for support from the Irish diaspora.

Lady Dudley contributed personally to the production of the annual reports of Lady Dudley's Scheme and presented them in an unusually pretty way. In the *Queen's Nurses' Magazine* 1904 it was observed that 'a Report is not generally a thing of beauty, but this one certainly is. The paper cover is white, tied with green ribbon, stamped with green letters, and the lovely little green badge which her nurses wear embossed upon it. There are several delightful photographs of the nurses at work, and views of their districts.[13]

This was a very inventive method of reaching the heart and purse strings of prospective subscribers. Additionally, the annual reports visually portrayed the Jubilee nurse at work and demonstrated the absolute poverty in these districts. The reports were accompanied by a map of the west of Ireland highlighting the district each nurse was located in. The committee of Lady Dudley's Scheme expressed concern in its annual report in 1912 regarding the cost of printing such high-quality and attractively presented reports. It was suggested that perhaps they should not be contained in 'so attractive a dress' and that a less expensive form of report might be adopted.[14] However, it was decided that the prestige of the elaborate productions attracted a more financially secure benefactor and increased the amount of financing received. Accordingly, the reports continued to be presented in an attractive fashion.

This use of public relations continued when the International Exhibition opened in Dublin in 1907. The committee of Lady

Dudley's Scheme made arrangements to display enlarged photographs of the districts in which the nurses worked and distributed literature in connection with the scheme.[15] The secretary of Lady Dudley's Scheme, Miss Myrrha Bradshaw, often acted as its in-house photographer. Lady Dudley, either alone or with officials from the Congested Districts Board, regularly visited patients and her nurses accompanied by Bradshaw, who would record such visits. Lord Dudley also made a tour of the poorest parts of Ireland with a view to establishing more district nurses.[16]

In her memoir *Seventy Years Young*, Lady Elizabeth Fingal remembered the Dudleys very fondly as being an enthusiastic, handsome and charming couple. On a routine visit to the Dudleys in Ireland, the Chancellor of the Exchequer was guided through the slums of Dublin and the poverty-stricken rural areas across Ireland and remarked: 'I did not know that in Western Europe such a country existed!'[17]

The committee of Lady Dudley's Scheme was hugely committed to the welfare of the nurses and aimed to communicate the nurses' work and appeal for continuing contributions on their behalf. Conrad Pim, the honorary secretary of the committee until 1957, was a very efficient and effective representative. He spoke at the Dublin Rotary Club meeting in the Metropole restaurant in 1935 about 'Nursing in the West' and gave a very informative and frank address. His statistics demonstrate the extent of the work of the Lady Dudley's nurses: the scheme employed 45 nurses who conducted 110,870 visits in the year 1934 alone. Most of the travel to these visits was done by bicycle over rough country terrain as Lady Dudley's Scheme could not afford the expense of motor cars.[18]

Pim very graciously left us a photographic legacy of every Lady Dudley Nurse outside her cottage in 1935.

CANDIDATES FOR NURSING IN THE SCHEME

In order for Lady Dudley's Scheme to succeed it relied completely on the quality and calibre of the nurses who would have to work in some of the most remote districts in Ireland. In 1903 Lady Dudley visited St Laurence's Nurses Home to meet the nurses she would be sending to the west of Ireland. In response to this visit, she is recorded as saying:

> In starting the scheme this spring it was felt that the chief factor upon which the working of it depended was the type of nurse selected for work in these districts. Everything depended on the nurse. Upon her character, tact, judgement and intelligence rested almost entirely the success or failure of the work which the committee desire to accomplish.[19]

It was hoped that these professional ladies would have a civilising and refining influence on the rural population and perhaps raise their expectations and standard of living, even though it was thought that the local population would be slow to accept the nurse's interference.

Many of the populations of these rural districts spoke only Irish and so it was necessary that nurses recruited under Lady Dudley's Scheme had some conversational Irish.

TRAINING

Each of the Jubilee nurses was fully trained – medically and surgically – and had completed district nursing training through the Queen's Institute. Those sent to the particularly rural areas under Lady Dudley's Scheme also required midwife certification. The nurses were visited and inspected at regular intervals by the superintendent of the Queen's Institute in Dublin, by different members of the Lady Dudley's Committee and by the inspector of the Congested Districts Board.[20] The districts to which these nurses were deployed were very scattered and isolated and this was highlighted in most of the early annual reports, which mention letters of praise, appeal and approval of the influence of the Jubilee nurses on the population. These reports vividly describe much of the hardship encountered by the nurses and feature many heart-rending accounts of individual cases attended and the difficulties in reaching some of their patients.

The committee made regular visits to the nurses to monitor their wellbeing, offer them encouragement and provide books and newspapers to keep them up to date with current affairs and to break the isolation. When the *Report of the Vice-Regal Commission on Poor Law Reform* in Ireland was published in 1906, it highly commended the work of the Jubilee nurses in the remote districts of Ireland and added:

> In our opinion the success of the Scheme for the Establishment of District Nurses in the poorest parts of Ireland is due very largely to the selection of highly-qualified nurses of experience and aptitude, with character and resource that enable them to discharge their lonely and laborious duty efficiently and with general satisfaction. These nurses have, we believe, gained the affection and respect of those they attend, and apart from the actual good they do to patients under the direction of the Dispensary Doctor, they are most useful advocates for sanitary conditions in the houses and surroundings of those with whom they come in contact.[21]

Because these districts were so isolated and lonely, and the workload so relentless, the committee of Lady Dudley's Scheme decided to limit the length of continuous residence in any district to three years.[22] Over time this changed and in some districts the nurses became longstanding members of their local community.

DEPARTURE OF LADY DUDLEY

Prior to the Earl and Lady Dudley's departure from Ireland in 1905, Lady Dudley visited her nurses in Annagry, Arranmore and Glengarriff and was encouraged by the success of their work and the service they were able to provide to the inhabitants of these distant places. In December a delegation of twelve of her nurses assembled to bid her a respectful farewell. They thanked Lady Dudley, and Nurse Elizabeth Cusack, who was one of the first appointed under the scheme, read the following address:

> Your Excellency – It is with the most sincere regret that we have assembled here to-day to bid you a respectful farewell upon your departure from Ireland. We wish to express our deep sense of gratitude for your great kindness to us since you founded 'The Lady Dudley Fund' for the establishment of district nurses in the poorest part of Ireland. Your frequent visits to the various remote districts in which we are stationed have greatly cheered us in our work, and stimulated us to renewed efforts on behalf of the poor of our districts. It has

been a great honour to us to work under your Excellency's wise and sympathetic guidance, and we can speak with intimate knowledge of how deeply grateful the people of those districts are for what you have done for them. We are quite unable to convey an adequate idea of the feeling of love and gratitude which has been inspired amongst these poor Western people by your Excellency's efforts for their welfare and aid in time of sickness. We are delighted to learn that your interest in the nursing scheme will not be lessened by your absence from Ireland, and that it is your intention from time to time to revisit the various centres where we are stationed, and can assure your Excellency that we shall continually look forward to your future visits with the keenest pleasure. May we ask your Excellency to do us the honour of accepting the accompanying cloak-clasp as a souvenir of our binding connection with your Excellency's nursing scheme, and we trust that your Excellency may long be spared to devote yourself to such useful and charitable work.

The gold cloak-clasp presented to Lady Dudley consisted of two linked Tara brooches. The brooches are reproductions of the Celtic ornament, the original of which is in the Kildare Street Museum, Dublin and is known as the 'Tara Brooch'. The brooches, which were set with Irish pearls from the River Slaney, had the names of the nurses inscribed on the back, and on the outside of the case is a little plaque, on which was engraved the nurses' badge.[23]

Upon her departure from Ireland as vicerine, Lady Dudley was succeeded by Lady Aberdeen as president of Lady Dudley's Scheme but remained a patron of the scheme until 1920. In the intervening years, Lady Dudley spent some time in Australia while her husband was stationed there as governor general between 1908 and 1911. During her time there, she attempted to establish a similar nursing scheme to the one in Ireland but faced a number of obstacles including opposition from the medical profession and sheer geographical adversity.

Between 1910 and 1914, Lady Dudley attempted to establish bush nursing orders throughout Australia. The Australian government eventually took over this concept of provision of nurses to isolated homes.

Lady Dudley drowned in a terrible accident on 26 June 1920. It was a Saturday morning when she arrived at their summer residence at Screebe Lodge, Rosmuck, County Galway, which is located on the shores of Camus Bay. Reports suggest that Lady Dudley, who was an excellent swimmer, went to bathe with her maid and while in the water collapsed and drowned. Her maid was unable to assist. Lady Dudley's body was recovered within half an hour and a doctor certified that her death was due to natural causes. The coroner for west Galway deemed it unnecessary to hold an inquest.[24] Lady Dudley was 53 and was buried at the Dudley family home on 3 July 1920.

The annual report of the committee of Lady Dudley's Scheme in 1920 lamented the loss of Lady Dudley in a short introductory paragraph, which ended: 'Those with whom she worked, those with whom she schemed, her Committee and her nurses all mourn the loss of a true friend and Benefactor to Ireland.'[25]

Reports of the tragic death were cabled around the world. Much was mentioned about Rachel Gurney and her life before marriage, about the difficulties the Dudleys had encountered in their marriage and subsequent separation, the lifestyle of the Earl of Dudley, his wealth and tax debts but very little regard was given to her contribution to district nursing. The Rachel Dudley who founded the nursing scheme in her name deserved recognition for her work and total commitment to strive for better conditions for the poor, for the education of women, and for the rights of women to work. Lady Dudley's Scheme was the poorer for the loss of its esteemed founder. Her lasting legacy to Ireland has only been acknowledged in the name of the scheme itself.

CONTINUANCE OF LADY DUDLEY'S SCHEME

Whenever a district became financially able to support and maintain its own nurse the committee of Lady Dudley's Scheme were relieved of this responsibility. The committee then granted all responsibility for a Jubilee nurse to her local district nursing association. The two districts of the Irish Homestead Association, a precursor of Lady Dudley's Scheme, were shortly taken over by them. This was the association Lady Dudley had referred to in her opening letter of appeal. The *Irish Homestead* was a newspaper devoted to Irish agricultural and industrial development and edited by George W. Russell. In 1901 it printed an article describing the benefits of the stationing of a Queen's nurse in rural communities. Readers quickly acted upon this information and subscriptions were raised and nurses allocated to several districts. The readers of the *Irish Homestead* who contributed towards funding these nurses effectively became a sort of district nursing association. They were then taken over by Lady Dudley's Scheme due to the location of the relevant districts of the west of Ireland.

Sometimes the services of the Lady Dudley's nurses were simply no longer required. In 1912, for instance, the committee of Lady Dudley's Scheme rejoiced when it closed the district of Foxford:

> ... Foxford no longer being classified as one of the poorest in the West of Ireland due to the enterprise and energy of the nuns of the Convent of Divine Providence, where the textile industry, initiated by them some years ago, is now a flourishing concern, providing employment to the poor inhabitants of the locality. The nursing work in this district consisted largely of maternity cases, and a fully qualified midwife was appointed by the Union.[26]

FUNDING OF LADY DUDLEY'S NURSING SCHEME

The scheme received funding from a number of outlets.

Government Grants

Under the Local Government Act 1925, the Irish government allocated funding to a series of schemes, including the School Medical Services Scheme, the County Tuberculosis Scheme and the Maternity and Child Welfare Scheme. These schemes required a qualified nurse for implementation in the various districts. In districts where there was no government-sponsored nurse to carry out these services, the Jubilee nurses undertook all of these duties. In the case of Lady Dudley's nurses, the committee of Lady Dudley's Scheme was paid a subvention by the government for each of its nurses who implemented such schemes. This relationship with the local government authorities of eight counties continued right through to the end of Lady Dudley's Scheme in 1974.

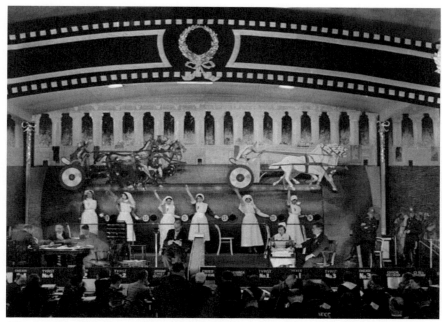

The funding of the Lady Dudley's Scheme was generally based on the dividends from the investment of capital generously donated. When the sweepstakes were set up, the Lady Dudley's Scheme was one of the organisations to benefit from grants issued by this organisation. Courtesy of the National Library of Ireland.

Hospitals' Sweepstakes

The Hospitals' Sweepstakes was a lottery system established in 1930 which was used to raise finances for Irish hospitals. The Queen's Institute began to receive much-needed financial support at this time from the Hospitals Commission, a government organisation responsible for the administration of the sweepstakes funds.

In 1932 a grant of £9,863 was paid from the November Handicap Sweepstakes and divided as follows: £5,000 was invested and constituted a part of the Endowment Fund with annual proceeds devoted to training of district nurses in the Irish Free State; £1,363 as a special subsidy fund to be invested and interest used for the purposes of helping districts that found it difficult to raise necessary funds; and £3,500 towards Lady Dudley's Scheme to be invested with an initial amount of £500 to open some districts immediately.[27] This funding continued for many years.

Passionate Plea for a Lady Dudley Nurse: Leenane Case Study

In 1939 the inhabitants of Leenane, County Galway wrote a heart-rending letter pleading for the provision of a Jubilee nurse to their community. The letter, all eleven pages of it, was signed by approximately 231 people and highlighted that it was the time she spent in Leenane with King Edward VII and Queen Alexandra which inspired Lady Dudley to found her nursing scheme. The letter promised a willingness on the part of the community to dedicate themselves to fundraising contributions to the cost of the nurse, with specific mention of their intention to run 'whist drives', dances or any other event that might assist. In its response, the committee of Lady Dudley's Scheme attributed a lack of funding to its inability to provide a nurse immediately but assured the people of Leenane that they would present their case to the Hospitals' Trust and the Department of Health.[28] A Queen's Institute affiliated nurse was never appointed to Leenane.

Patronage of Lady Dudley's Scheme

Lady Dudley's husband continued to be the patron of Lady Dudley's Scheme until his death in 1932 and his son the 3rd Earl of Dudley (William Humble Eric Ward) remained patron until his death in 1969. The Dudleys' eldest daughter, the Lady Morvyth Benson, acted as vice-president until her death in 1959. Similar family continuity occurred when members on the committee over the years were succeeded by their relatives and, in particular, their daughters. The headquarters of Lady Dudley's Scheme were originally located in the Viceregal Lodge before moving to 33 Molesworth Street, Dublin. In 1940 it moved to 48 Lower Leeson Street, Dublin 2, the same address as the Irish branch of the Queen's Institute. Both organisations moved to 19 Pembroke Park, Dublin 4 in 1965. The headquarters relocated on one final occasion in 1968 to 29 Leeson Street upon cessation of Queen's Institute training activities.

The Congested Districts Board Cottages

The Congested Districts Board was established in 1891 to alleviate the extreme poverty present in areas throughout the west of

Ireland where inhabitants lived in very close proximity to each other with virtually no income or resources. Lady Dudley's Scheme received contributions from the Congested Districts Board from its establishment. These contributions were initially provided in the form of rent and furnishings in each of five districts. By 1905, the board had consented to build five more nurses' cottages as additional districts were established.[29] Under the Labourers Act 1906, a sum of £4,250,000 was allocated by the British government for loans to rural authorities in Ireland for the construction of housing, repayable in 68½ years by annual instalments of 3.25 per cent, covering principal and interest.[30] The Congested Districts Board, upon receipt of a portion of this fund, charged Lady Dudley's Scheme a low rate of interest on the capital outlay of its cottages.[31] Some of the railway and steamship companies also offered to carry furniture and stores destined for the nurses free of charge.[32]

Cottages that were built for Lady Dudley's nurses became a problem for the committee towards the end of the scheme due to questions over ownership, rents due and maintenance. The cottages were very basic and became more and more dilapidated over time. The living conditions of the nurses was an important consideration for the committee so the provision of running water, electricity and maintenance became an extraordinary expense as the buildings depreciated in condition.

CESSATION OF QUEEN'S INSTITUTE OPERATIONS AND THE CONTINUANCE OF LADY DUDLEY'S SCHEME THEREAFTER

As discussed in Chapter 2, the Queen's Institute ceased the training of nurses in 1968. As in the case of all district nursing associations previously affiliated with the Queen's Institute during its existence, Lady Dudley's Scheme was capable of continuing to operate independently, using funds which it raised itself.

Miss Delaney, former inspector of the Queen's Institute, was welcomed to the staff and committee of Lady Dudley's Scheme as a supervisor/inspector upon her departure from the Queen's Institute in 1968. Lady Dudley's Scheme still had 33 nurses and one nurse in training for district work with An Bord Altranais.[33] Over the next few years Lady Dudley's Scheme maintained the 33 districts. In 1970 Lord Dudley passed away and the committee of Lady Dudley's Scheme expressed sympathy with the Earl of Dudley upon the death of his father. The original scheme conceived by his mother in 1903 had expanded from just two nurses at its inception to 49 districts at the height of its existence across Donegal, Mayo, Galway, Sligo, Roscommon, Kerry, Cork and Cavan. Upon its closure in 1974, Lady Dudley's Scheme still maintained 33 districts, independent from the support of the Queen's Institute.

This paragraph is from the Final Report (covering 1 January 1973 to 31 March 1974) – by Gladys McConnell, Chairman of Lady Dudley's Scheme.

> The Committee of Lady Dudley's Nursing Scheme presents the Seventy-first and Final Report. In many ways it has been a very successful year. It has also been a sad year.
>
> On the 1st April 1974 we passed our Nursing responsibility to the Department of Health, and our assets, after all debts and financial commitments be deducted, to The Commissioners of Charitable Donations and Requests.
>
> The reason for this change is to be found in the ideal of National responsibility. The sick poor in the remote districts and islands of Ireland are no longer the concern of a few charitably-minded people, but, rather the responsibility of the whole country.[34]

Lady Aberdeen and the Women's National Health Association

An important spark in the evolution of district nursing associations throughout Ireland was the arrival of Ishbel Marjoribanks – Lady Aberdeen, Countess of Temaire and wife of the viceroy of Ireland from 1906 to 1914. Born in 1857, Lady Aberdeen had homes in Scotland and in London's Grosvenor Square, and a country house outside London after her marriage to Lord Aberdeen. As supporters of Gladstone and home rule for Ireland, the Aberdeens spent a total of ten years in Ireland through two visits as viceroys. Their first, in 1886, lasted for six months and was marked by Lady Aberdeen's interest in developing cottage industries such as lace-making that would benefit rural Irish families directly. She set up the Irish Home Industries Association to assist in this endeavour.

Lady Aberdeen also coordinated the Irish Village at the World's Fair in Chicago in 1893. It was one of the main financial successes of the exhibition and £20,000 worth of Irish goods was sold.[35]

Lady Aberdeen began her involvement with district nursing as a new bride in the village of Tarves on the family estate in Scotland in the late 1870s when the Aberdeens set up a cottage hospital with doctor and district nurse as a free service to their tenants.[36] In 1889 she was a committee member of the first council of the Queen's Institute of Scotland.[37]

After moving to Canada with her husband as governor general in 1893, Lady Aberdeen founded the Victorian Order of Nurses for Canada in 1897. This non-profit organisation provides, to this day, a vast range of health services to Canadian communities. It began in a similar way to the Jubilee nurses in Ireland, offering prenatal education, baby clubs, school health services and visiting nursing and coordinated homecare programmes. The organisation has expanded its activities, setting up hospitals, offering home-based palliative care, foot-care clinics, respite care, primary health-care at women's shelters for children and youth at risk and many more invaluable services. A total of 75 different programmes are provided by 4,500 healthcare workers and 9,016 community volunteers. Its website proudly proclaims Lady Aberdeen as founder and announces that the 'Victorian Order of Nurses Canada will

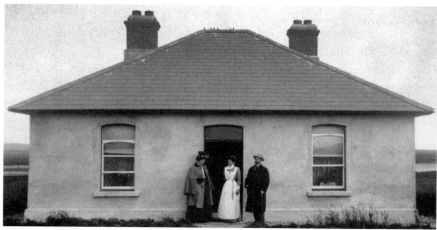

Lord and Lady Aberdeen with the nurse at Geesala, 1906–1914.
Courtesy of the National Library of Ireland.

continue to be a dynamic and responsive community-based organisation working with local people everywhere to help identify healthcare needs and develop appropriate services'.[38]

It was on her return to Ireland in 1906 that the scourge of tuberculosis, known also as consumption or the white plague, became Lady Aberdeen's personal crusade. Health statistics in Ireland made for horrendous reading, as tuberculosis was a killer primarily of young people between the ages of 15 and 35. Sixteen per cent of deaths in the country were caused by tuberculosis. As will be described in the case studies in Chapter 6, there was also a great deal of superstition and ignorance about the disease. In the days before antibiotics, prevention of the spread of the disease was vital.

In 1924 Lady Aberdeen recalled all the activities of the earlier period in 'Health and Happiness in the Homes of Ireland', an article she wrote for *The Voice of Ireland*, a collection of articles contributed by leading members of Irish society. She organised lectures, demonstrations and a travelling exhibition, based on the itinerant tuberculosis exhibition in the United States. 'Travelling caravans were fitted out to reach remote districts where there were no halls big enough for the show,' she wrote. There were two caravans – 'Éire', the first, was to burn down but it was replaced by 'Phoenix' and 'Bluebird'. The staff were selected so that they could include dancing and singing in the show, 'providing the lighter side to the lectures and health talks'. The Gaelic League was asked to provide an Irish-speaking lecturer for the west of Ireland, who was supplied with lantern slides and Gaelic literature to aid the presentation of valuable information.[39]

In 1908, Lady Aberdeen sent two nurses to Edinburgh to study the most up-to-date information on tuberculosis. They were then placed in Dublin, one on the north side of the city and one on the south, and were called the Tuberculosis Queen's Nurses. Following a recommendation from a doctor in one of the ten hospitals in the scheme, they visited patients who were afflicted with TB. Their clients were both male and female, of all ages, mostly underprivileged, and were advised on ventilation, hygiene, diet and isolation from the rest of the family, if possible. These nurses assisted where they could to get clean lodgings away from tenements, and a Samaritan Fund was used to provide better nourishment. Visiting twice a week, they often had to recommend dying patients be sent to 'the Union Hospital or one of the homes for the dying'.[40]

Newcastle Sanatorium, now Peamount Hospital, was founded in 1912 by Lady Aberdeen's Woman's National Health Association and was funded by a government grant of £25,000 following the Health Insurance Act of 1911. Lady Aberdeen was also instrumental in the establishment of a tuberculosis dispensary in Charles Street, Dublin; a holiday home in Sutton on the north coast of Dublin which was referred to as a 'preventorium'; and the Alan A. Ryan Home-Hospital for Advanced Cases. Sanatoria and their development was seen as important in the treatment and prevention of TB at the time and for many decades after but were not always welcomed into communities due to a fear of the disease.

Lady Aberdeen's support for the Jubilee nurses was undeniable. She took over the Lady Dudley Committee on her reinstatement as viceroy's wife and in 1912 was appointed honorary president of the Irish branch of the Queen's Institute.

An interesting aspect of the propaganda associated with many of the projects that Lady Aberdeen was involved in was the use of nationalist motifs. She was acutely aware that her message would need support from all elements of the community if it was to be successful. In terms of political views, as a friend of Gladstone and later a supporter of John Redmond she believed in home rule for Ireland. In 'Sorrows of Ireland' (1916) she deplores the English rule and their misunderstanding that led to a police and civil service with 'a supreme sense of responsibility to the British Treasury rather than what is needed for the health of the people of Ireland and the development of the country's resources'.[41] Her views and actions were often not understood. As representative of the crown in Ireland she was the focus of much negative comment and unfair criticism of being duplicitous or naive. She energetically pursued her goals 'in the face of apathy rooted in historic causes'.[42] One of these aims was to improve living standards through the influence of women in the home.

In 1893 Lady Aberdeen became the first president of the International Council of Women, whose inaugural meeting was held in Washington DC in 1888. It began with nine countries which met nationally every three years and internationally every five years. Today, it is composed of 70 countries and is a highly influential organisation within the United Nations. Lady Aberdeen's belief in the power of women as a force for positive change in society expressed itself in the formation of an organisation called the Women's National Health Association.[43]

WOMEN'S NATIONAL HEALTH ASSOCIATION OF IRELAND

In a flurry of articles in national and local newspapers in 1907, Lady Aberdeen presented the objectives of the Women's National Health Association to the people of Ireland. This was to 'arouse public opinion, and especially that of the women of Ireland, to a sense of their responsibility regarding the public health, and to spread the knowledge of what may be done in every home and by every householder to guard against disease and to promote the upbringing of a healthy vigorous race'.[44] The health problems under consideration were tuberculosis, infantile mortality (responsible at the time for 95 of every 1,000 deaths), and milk supply

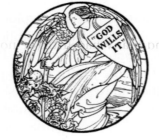

WOMEN'S NATIONAL HEALTH ASSOCIATION OF IRELAND.

Objects.

1. To arouse public opinion, and especially that of the Women of Ireland, to a sense of responsibility regarding the public health.

2. To spread the knowledge of what may be done in every home, and by every householder, to guard against disease, and to eradicate it when it appears.

3. To promote the upbringing of a healthy and vigorous race.

Card of Membership held by _____

_____ Branch

_____ Local President

Ishbel Aberdeen
President of Association.

Courtesy of the National Archives of Ireland, Peamount Collection.

(before pasteurisation, milk was responsible for the spread of many diseases such as typhoid, typhus, scarlet fever and smallpox).

Lady Aberdeen also outlined how the association planned to disseminate information:

> The methods whereby information may be spread and action initiated will readily suggest themselves, namely 1. Popular lectures and meetings on health subjects by medical men and others. 2. Simple health talks with small circles of working mothers. 3. The appointment of women health officers, health visitors and sanitary inspectors. 4. The urging of sanitary questions on the attention of local authorities. 5. The compiling and general distribution of simple health leaflets and other health literature. 6. The teaching of hygiene and of domestic science in every school. 7. The appointment of district nurses in districts where such are not already working.[45]

While district nurses were last on the list of methods to be employed by the association, they proved to be the most enduring. By 1910, there were 155 branches of the Women's National Health Association.[46] Thirty-eight branches eventually had an affiliated nurse, and many of these evolved into district nursing associations which lasted well over 60 years.

The existence of the Women's National Health Association had the important side effect of providing a socially respectable and fashionable system of governance for the operation of many district nursing associations. Women at that time were often deprived of further education by social mores and many had little or no business or work experience. Enthusiastic members of the Women's National Health Association were introduced to financial responsibilities, meetings protocol, annual reports and supervision of staff and volunteers.

Women were offered practical advice by the president of the association, Lady Aberdeen, in a twenty-page pamphlet printed and distributed by the Women's National Health Association. *Organisation of Local Branches* sets out in clear, precise detail the way in which a new branch of the association should be organised. The date of publication is not clear but it may have been 1913, the year of incorporation of the Women's National Health Association at 9 Ely Place in Dublin.[47] This pamphlet is important because it is a blueprint for most of the district nursing associations set up all over Ireland under affiliation with the Queen's Institute. It begins by explaining how to organise a new branch of the association and advises that one should initially privately consult and gain the support of all representative women, the leading clergy, the medical men and the local authorities in the neighbourhood. When there is consensus among '*all classes and all creeds* to unite in the one aim of promoting the public health of the community by every possible means' (emphasis added), provisional officers should be assigned. A public inaugural meeting should then be organised and 'every effort should be made to make it as representative as possible, including in the invitation both ladies and gentlemen'. A number of pages describe how a voluntary committee should conduct itself with regard to the posts of president, vice-president, honorary secretary, honorary treasurer and members of working committees. Lady Aberdeen advises that branch districts should correspond to the dispensary districts. If a dispensary nurse is not already present, one should be obtained from the Queen's Institute.

Lady Aberdeen also suggested methods of publicising the aims and work of each new branch of the Women's National Health Association. Professionally printed publicity material was advised. Membership cards for the association had been designed by Miss Purser and Miss Elvery of Dublin and were available in both Irish and English. One could also have a blue and saffron Celtic-designed badge instead of a membership card but this required payment of a penny each. The badge could be purchased in enamel and gilt for 3s 6d or enamel and silver at 4s each.

A large part of this memorandum set out the elements of Lady Aberdeen's campaign for the eradication of tuberculosis. It includes advice on the establishment of Samaritan funds, tuberculosis dispensaries and garden shelters for infectious patients. The main emphasis was on education, as it was with the Queen's Institute.

Infant mortality was also a subject of much concern for Lady Aberdeen. The dissemination of information regarding the rearing, feeding and general management of infants among young girls and young mothers was vital. Nurses or health visitors urged for the establishment of schools and babies' clubs for mothers. These babies' clubs were successful and many were still in existence until the late 1940s. They distributed vital supplementary vitamins through the 'Emergency', when the numbers subscribing to the clubs increased greatly as the poor suffered inability to purchase food due to inflation and shortages.[48]

Care of school children and their health was another interest of Lady Aberdeen. Efforts were made to get the National Education Commissioners to encourage a break for children during the school day and to provide subsidised meals or cocoa and milk. Branches of the Girls' Guild of Good Health and the Boys' National Health Battalion could be set up on application to the literature secretary of the Viceregal Lodge. Petitions and resolutions in favour of extending the system of medical inspection of schools to Ireland were drawn up and sent to politicians and relevant government departments. Open-air schools were encouraged.

Finally, according to the aforementioned memorandum, mothers who were members of the Women's National Health Association 'should be urged to make it a point of honour to teach their children habits of health, cleanliness, and self-control'.

This list is intriguing and includes briefly:

(a) Daily ablutions including cleaning of teeth;
(b) Proper and thorough mastication of food explaining the evils that come from bolting meals;
(c) Care as to cleanliness and neatness in clothing especially underclothing;
(d) Self-control in not eating and drinking between meals or whenever inclined. It is not a good plan to give sweeties to children at all sorts of odd times, or to let them take a swill of water whenever inclined;
(e) To breathe through the nose and not through the mouth;
(f) Not to rake or make stewed tea, explaining to them how tea which has been long drawn is poison;
(g) To send them to bed early.

The ladies of the Women's National Health Association were encouraged to sustain smaller agricultural industries including gardening, poultry and bee-keeping. Good financial control was also vital. One third of each annual subscription was to be sent to the Central Council for organisation purposes. The Central Council for the Women's National Health Association was formed by representatives from branches of the association and met during the Dublin Spring Show as railway fares were reduced at that time. A printed annual report was expected from every branch.[49]

SLÁINTE

Sláinte, translated as 'good health', was a monthly journal produced by the Women's National Health Association. It was edited, and many of the articles were written, by Lady Aberdeen herself. Her style of writing was emphatic and did not seem to understand the fatalistic view of those caught in the unrelenting poverty trap in Ireland, rural and urban, of the period. The goals of her project, so directly enunciated in *Sláinte*, would prove to be a politically difficult task to set for the new members of her association. The magazine was produced very professionally on glossy paper, with lots of photographs, by the publishers Maunsel and Company of Abbey Street, Dublin. Much of the advertising space was dedicated to health-related subjects such as baby foods, soap, disinfectants and patented medicines, while Switzers and other ladies' outfitters also availed of the opportunity to advertise. Rural readers were targeted with ads for milk cans and strainers, seeds and tools. The first edition of *Sláinte* was published in January 1909 and could be purchased for a penny.

In May 1909, a report on the second annual meeting of the Women's National Health Association, which had taken place in the beautiful lecture hall of the Royal Dublin Society at Leinster House (now Dáil Éireann), featured in *Sláinte*. Every month a selection of reports and letters from the branches around the country were published, with upbeat accounts of successful and novel fundraising events which nearly always occurred 'despite the inclement weather'. An example of a district report from March 1912 – 'Six Weeks at the Bray Babies Club' – describes the work done from 1 January to 12 February. There were 44 new cases – 'three babies died but all the others have done well'. The formation of a sewing guild from a committee of ladies associated with several branches was described. An initial donation from the president of the association to buy fabric was used to sew garments for babies to be distributed to the poor in the area. Clean milk distribution was also discussed in the short article.

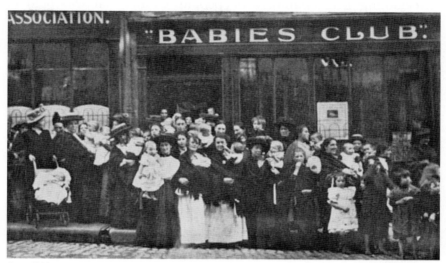

From a photo] [taken by Lady Aberdeen

ST. MONICA'S BABIES' CLUB, DUBLIN.

Opened in St. Augustine Street, in June, by the Dublin Branch of the W.N.H.A.

St Monica's Baby Club, June 1909. Courtesy of the National Library of Ireland.

New branches and babies' clubs were always welcomed by the organisation. The magazine remained focused on health issues and articles on tuberculosis and other diseases were published, many from medical and nursing journals. Reports on similar work to that being carried out by the Women's National Health Association came from Canada (where the Victorian Order of Nurses was successfully established by Lady Aberdeen), the US, England, France and Switzerland, where the concept of sanatoria had developed. In September 1910 Lady Plunket gave an account of New Zealand's struggle with infant mortality. She discussed the development and training of 'Plunket Nurses' to visit babies and teach mothers on proper care for infants.

1911 was a big year for *Sláinte* because of Uí Breasail, an exhibition of health issues organised by the Women's National Health Association. It involved sideshow stalls from a number of branches which demonstrated produce from districts throughout Ireland. Lady Aberdeen was deeply committed to the concept of international trade fairs which, at the height of success in mid-Victorian times, were still an influential way of informing and entertaining great numbers of people. Uí Breasail was held in Ballsbridge, Dublin for two weeks from 24 May to 7 June 1911. It was a combination of carnival – featuring entertainment and a large restaurant – and education, with stands on district nursing, tuberculosis prevention (the caravan), healthy eating, home cleanliness, and a large literature stall. *Sláinte* began 1911 with a calendar advertising the exhibition. The central image was of the interior of a cottage of domestic bliss titled 'a scene from the village in "Uí Breasail"'. They also published a souvenir edition to commemorate Uí Breasail in May.

By 1914, concerns were focused on the 'war in Europe' and the Women's National Health Association, Red Cross and St John's Ambulance cooperated to set up work parties to make shirts and comforts for soldiers at the front. *Sláinte* was last published in January 1915 and the Aberdeens left Ireland the following month. Lady Aberdeen had effectively monopolised the magazine herself and there was no successor to continue the work. It was never financially self-supporting and included constant reminders to subscribers to try and spread the word among new readers. *Sláinte*, 'our little fairy', was important because it reminded the 'workers that they were part of a great army, calling on all to join in the crusade against all enemies of Ireland's good health'.

DEMISE OF THE WOMAN'S NATIONAL HEALTH ASSOCIATION

Gradually, branches of the Women's National Health Associations dropped the name and evolved into, simply, 'district nursing associations'. The reasons for this are varied but one factor may have been the foundation of the United Irishwomen. In 1895, under the presidency of Sir Horace Plunkett, the Irish Agricultural Organisation Society was founded as a central body for agricultural cooperatives. With its support, Anita Lett, an Englishwoman living in Wexford, founded the United Irishwomen in 1911. Lady Aberdeen and the Women's National Health Association initially welcomed this group but members quickly realised that the aims and the territories of the two organisations were too similar not to find themselves in competition, particularly in rural areas.[50] A public controversy erupted in 1912 following a decision by the United Irishwomen to provide health visitors, who were not hospital-trained nurses, into their districts. Seen as second-grade nurses, they were not in a position to contest the Jubilee nurse service offered by the Women's National Health Association.[51] The overall battle, however, was lost as the Women's National Health Association was highly dependent on Lady Aberdeen as a driving force and suffered enormously upon her departure. The United Irishwomen became, in 1935, the Irish Country Women's Association, which is still a thriving educational and social support organisation for women all over Ireland.

By 1942 the Women's National Health Association had become a cluster of 'babies' clubs' and Peamount Hospital, based in 9 Ely Place, Dublin. The contribution of these babies' clubs cannot be overlooked and they were still a force in 1942. The report of the Central Babies Club Committee that year showed 81,302 attendances at the nine clubs in the Dublin area. They offered food and vitamin supplements and cod liver oil. Lectures were given by a health visitor in addition to classes in cooking, dancing, sewing and knitting. Cheap dentures were available for mothers. At Christmas there was access to the Mansion House fuel fund and government departments provided supplies to the needy of tea, sugar and butter.[52]

In 1962, the Women's National Health Association ceased to exist in its own right, becoming Peamount Hospital Incorporated. The contribution made by it, and Lady Aberdeen, to the system of domiciliary nursing care by Jubilee nurses is a subtle one. By teaching the principles of organisation, basic business skills and the importance of health to women across all facets of Irish society, Lady Aberdeen instilled the acumen necessary to develop a network of successful district nursing associations throughout the country.

NOTES

1   Lady Dudley's Scheme for Establishment of Nurses in Poorest Parts of Ireland (hereafter the Lady Dudley's Scheme), 1904, p. 6. National Library, Dublin.

2   The West of Ireland Association, 1st Annual Report 1900. National Library, Dublin.

3   Chris Cunneen, 'Dudley, Lady Rachel (1867–1920)', *Australian Dictionary of Biography*, vol. 8 (Melbourne: Melbourne University Press, 1981. Online edition available at: http://www.abd.anu.au/biography-dudley-lady-rachel-6376 [Accessed 6 August 2012].

4   *New York Times*, 28 June 1920. Available at: http://www.query.nytimes.com/gst/abstract.html?res=F20C14FC3E5E1B728DDDA10A94DE405B808EF1D3# [Accessed 6 August 2012].

5   Amanda R. Andrews, 'The Great Ornamentals: New Vice-Regal Women and their Imperial Work, 1884–1914', unpublished thesis, University of Western Sydney, 2002.

6   Lady Dudley's Scheme, 3rd Annual Report, April 1905–6, p. 16. National Library, Dublin.

7   *Weekly Irish Times*, 11 August 1903, p. 13. Irish Times Archives.

8   Lady Dudley's Scheme, 1st Annual Report, 1903–4, p. 8. National Library, Dublin.

9   Ibid., p. 5.

10   Ibid., pp. 10, 14.

11   Ibid., p. 5.

12   Ibid., p. 12.

13   *Queen's Nurses' Magazine* (September 1904), p. 30. The Queen's Nursing Institute, London.

14   Lady Dudley's Scheme, 9th Annual Report, 1912, p. 1. National Library, Dublin.

15   Lady Dudley's Scheme, 4th Annual Report, 1906, p. 16. National Library, Dublin.

16   *Queen's Nurses' Magazine* (September 1904), p. 31. The Queen's Nursing Institute, London.

17   Elizabeth, Countess of Fingall, *Seventy Years Young: Memoirs of Elizabeth Countess of Fingall* (Dublin: The Lilliput Press, 1937), pp. 281, 282.

18   Address by Mr C. Pim, Dublin Rotary Club, Irish Times, 3 September 1935. Department of Health files, A/128/16. National Archives, Dublin.

19   *Weekly Irish Times*, 12 December 1903, p. 5. Irish Times Archives.

20   Lady Dudley's Scheme, 1st Annual Report, 1903–4, p. 3. National Library, Dublin.

21   *Irish Rural Life and Industry in Connection with Irish International Exhibition 1907* (catalogue), pp. 276, 277. Royal Dublin Society Library, Dublin.

22   Lady Dudley's Scheme, 9th Annual Report, 1912, p. 10. National Library, Dublin.

23   *Queen's Nurses' Magazine* (December 1905), pp. 93, 94. The Queen's Nursing Institute, London.

24   *New York Times*, 28 June 1920, p. 1. Available at http://www.query.nytimes.com/gst/abstract.html?res=F20C14FC3E5E1B728DDDA10A94DE405B808EF1D3# [Accessed 6 August 2012].

25   Lady Dudley's Scheme, Annual Report, 1920. National Library, Dublin.

26   Lady Dudley's Scheme, 9th Annual Report, 1912, p. 12. National Library, Dublin.

27   Letter from Department of Local Government and Public Health to QIDN, 1 March 1932. Department of Health files, M104/100. National Archives, Dublin. Under the Public Hospitals Act 1933, the Minister for Health was empowered to make grants out of the now legalised Hospitals Trust Fund to any organisation which had for its sole or principal object the provision of nurses. The only organisation at the time which was eligible to receive these funds was the Queen's Institute of District Nursing. When the QIDN made further request for funds, the Hospitals Commission felt that 'whilst there is no doubt that the Irish Branch of the Queen's Institute has, in view of its limited financial resources, done very praiseworthy work in regard to the provision of District Nursing for the sick poor, the Country generally cannot be said to possess a really efficient or co-ordinated nursing service.' They continue that 'there would appear to be a good case for a reorganisation on a national basis of the whole nursing service in the state'.

28   Lady Dudley's Scheme, Department of Health files, A128/16. National Archives, Dublin.

29   Lady Dudley's Scheme, 3rd Annual Report, 1905–6, p. 12. National Library, Dublin.

30   *Irish Rural Life and Industry in Connection with Irish International Exhibition 1907*, p. 281. Royal Dublin Society Library, Dublin.

31   Lady Dudley's Scheme, 1st Annual Report, 1905–6, p. 12. National Library, Dublin.

32   *Queen's Nurses' Magazine* (July 1905), p. 53. The Queen's Nursing Institute, London.

33   Lady Dudley's Scheme, Annual Report, 1968, P.48/3(7), Donegal Archives, Lifford, Co. Donegal.

34   Ibid.

35   Maureen Keane, *Ishbel: Lady Aberdeen in Ireland* (Newtownards: Colourpoint Books, 1999).

36   Ibid.

37   Florence Nightingale, 'Introduction', in William Rathbone, *The History and Progress of District Nursing* (London: Macmillan, 1890).

38   Victorian Order of Nurses Canada, official website information, www.von. ca [accessed 27 August 2012].

39   Marchioness of Aberdeen, 'Health and Happiness in the Homes of Ireland', in William G. Fitzgerald (ed.), *The Voice of Ireland* (Dublin: John Heywood Ltd, 1924).

40   *Queen's Nurses' Magazine* (December 1908). The Queen's Nursing Institute, London.

41   Ishbel, Lady Aberdeen, *The Sorrows of Ireland* (Cambridge, 1916). National Library, Dublin.

42 Marchioness of Aberdeen, 'Health and Happiness in the Homes of Ireland'.

43 Keane, *Ishbel: Lady Aberdeen in Ireland.*

44 Lady Aberdeen, press cuttings, February–March 1907. Peamount Hospital Collection, National Archives, Dublin.

45 *Sláinte*, journal for the Women's National Health Association (WNHA). Complete set available in the Peamount Hospital Collection, National Archives, Dublin.

46 Ibid.

47 *Organisation of Local Branches*, pamphlet for the WNHA. Peamount Hospital Collection, National Archives, Dublin.

48 Annual reports of the WNHA Baby Clubs. Peamount Hospital Collection, National Archives, Dublin.

49 *Organisation of Local Branches.*

50 Keane, *Ishbel: Lady Aberdeen in Ireland.*

51 *Irish Times*, 6 June 1913, Report on the first Council of Nurses. Irish Times Archives.

52 WNHA annual reports. Peamount Hospital Collection, National Archives, Dublin.

CHAPTER 6

Case Studies of the Jubilee Nurses

An important element of the story of the Jubilee nurses is that of their patients. Understanding the great human difficulties and triumphs of patients which formed such a large part of the daily routine of the nurses illuminates their lives immensely. Accounts of the nurses' work were sent by the Lady Dudley's nurses to head office to be used in the propaganda that was essential to the establishment and continuation of the scheme. The accounts are heart-rending in their bleakness. These descriptions of the hardship suffered in the west of Ireland were useful in loosening the purse strings of the wealthy benefactors to Lady Dudley's Scheme. We have selected a very small number of these letters to illuminate different aspects of the work. They were not fictional and the authenticity of the plight of the people is supported by independent commentators at the time, namely the Congested Districts Board.

A fundraising device which was regularly employed involved the publication in newspapers of an account of 'a day in the life' of the Jubilee nurse. These observations, recorded by an independent commentator who would accompany the nurse around the district, showed the extraordinary variety of cases covered. They also emphasise the enormous commitment of the nurse in her efforts to reach everyone, no matter how long it made her day. Some nurses wrote letters to head office with stories and sample cases that would be of interest to their peers. The *Queen's Nurses' Magazine* published them monthly. The poverty of patients became less extreme with time but the comfort and care offered by the nurses to people in their own homes did not diminish. The gratitude expressed by patients to the nurses also remained consistent. A nurse naming herself as 'Fuzzy Wuzzy' in an anonymous contribution to the

Queen's Nurses' Magazine in December 1904 described the disturb-
ing poverty and hardship which she encountered in her district
in the west of Ireland, and also the reluctance of the people to
abandon their belief in old customs and the fairies. She went on
to say:

> There are, I venture to say, few houses where the nurse is not welcome.
> How delighted they are to have someone to meet them in a friendly
> way and show them what to do, and not only show them, but do what
> is necessary, and, as they say themselves, not to have a 'disgust' at the
> sick person. Their gratitude is beautiful to see, and their expressions
> of thanks so warm that at times I feel humbled and ashamed of having
> done so little for them.[1]

SUPERSTITION

According to nurses in the early stages of their mission, their overwhelming concern was the uphill battle to overcome the prevalence
of superstition, 'handy women' and the traders of charms and
potions. A huge fear among their patients of change, and particularly of hospitals, required an all-absorbing energy and dedication
to overcome by the nurses. It was necessary for them to win the
trust of the people and to turn them away from dangerous practices.

Describing this resistance to change, a nurse in the west of
Ireland wrote in 1904: '… and though the patient may feel more
comfortable and more cheerful while I am there, when I am gone
the "knowledgeable" women talk it over and say such a thing was
never done before, and they hope it will be all right, but they don't
think it will, it is no wonder that sometimes the patient is worried
to death'.[2] Nurse Hedderman in the Aran Islands remarked in 1917
that 'one of my chief difficulties in connection with nursing, in fact
the greatest obstacle I had to surmount in the early days, was the
native aversion to doctors, as well as everything associated with
medicine in any form. The dispensary they regarded as a kind of
guillotine or death trap – a tribunal from which, if they entered,
they were never to emerge.'[3]

A Lady Dudley nurse reported in 1908 of this fear of doctors
which resulted in great suffering for one of her young patients.

A patient living 9 miles away, 13 years old, fell off a donkey and broke his leg. They sent for a bone setter, who bound the leg round very tightly with little sticks. The priest called and asked me to go and see them. I found leg very swollen and child in great pain. After talking to them for about 3 quarters of an hour I at last persuaded them to let me cut them off. Placed leg in padded crinkled cardboard, and told them to send for doctor to set it properly. Visited them several times since, but they won't get the doctor.[4]

It was still a problem in 1935 in Donegal. The nurses in Fanad district worried about the 'people who make quite a trade selling charms and herbal concoctions'. Describing the results of the neglect which arose from a dependency on these mystical remedies, Nurse Clancy said: 'One man who had a septic finger was terrified that a doctor would operate, so he bought a plaster from one of these men, which he wore for nearly a month. The poison, of course, spread, and in the end he had to go to a doctor, and he lost his finger, and very nearly his arm as well.'[5]

INJURIES AND DRESSINGS

On 15 September 1905 a Lady Dudley nurse sent in her report, giving a brief description of her life, as requested by Lady Dudley.

I am quite ready for a holiday. I have been very busy for the past eight weeks — nearly all surgical cases. At present I have six bad surgical cases on. I have one six miles from me in one direction, and another seven miles off in the opposite direction. The others I can take 'en route'. The distances here certainly are very great. I have a dear wee child on at present. She was fearfully burned. Poor wee pet is only 4½ years old. It is four weeks to-morrow since it happened. She has been so good, I thought she should be rewarded, so I sent away for a doll for her and dressed it as an 'Irish Colleen'. The poor child had never possessed a doll before, and it was most touching to see her delight. She caressed it and made such a fuss. The next day I visited the child and enquired after Dollie. The poor child was in a terrible state. She said her Dollie would surely die as it could not eat anything or drink any milk and she was sure it never went to sleep. September 19th — I received a call, so had to leave this until now. I have been out the last three nights, and have not had a chance to send it off until now.[6]

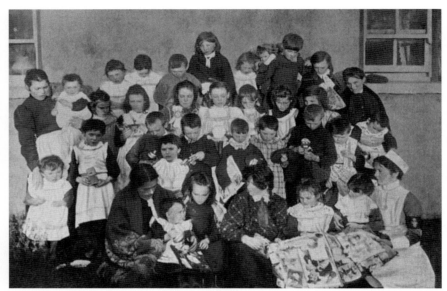

Toys and small gifts were collected all over Ireland and sent to the nurses of the
Lady Dudley's Scheme for distribution at Christmas.
Courtesy of the National Library of Ireland.

Another child patient for whom the doll was a great help was
described in 1911. It was tradition for the Lady Dudley's Committee
to organise the sending of toys for Christmas to every district.

> I had this month a very severe case of scalding: patient a little girl
> aged five. I do not know how I would have managed the dressings as
> her screams were awful, but for the doll and a ball taken from the box
> of toys so kindly sent.[7]

In 1904 a nurse from Galway wrote to the *Queen's Nurses' Magazine*
deploring the struggle to inform the people of first-aid care.

> Nurse has a dreadful case on her hands at present. A man here gashed
> his knee with a hatchet. To stop the bleeding his mother applied pig's
> manure! The doctor took an hour to cleanse the wound, but even so
> the result has been blood poisoning and the man is still very ill indeed.[8]

A Lady Dudley nurse reported in 1906:

> A deaf and dumb man who walked in six miles to have his arms dressed.
> When I went to him he pointed to his arms in the most pathetic way
> to show me they were sore. He had several carbuncles or large boils on

them. I cleansed and dressed them every day and they were quite well in ten days, which pleased him very much.[9]

In 1908 the infection of a patient was fatal and very distressing:

Another patient whose cabin is 21 miles off. I was called up at 12 o'clock by doctor and asked if I would go and attend a patient who was suffering from acute blood poisoning and was very delirious. I stayed until 4 o'clock and left her sleeping. Doctor made an incision into arm. A doctor from a neighbouring town was sent for, but arrived too late to do any good. She died on the 4th May.[10]

A disease such as breast cancer still takes lives today but most women detect it early and there are comprehensive and effective ways of treating it. When these fail, there are real ways to alleviate the suffering and pain. Such a scenario was very different in 1896 when there were no painkillers or sedatives to assist in palliative care. A nurse in St Patrick's Home took a tram to visit a patient in an outlying district.

Cancer of the breast – a young woman of 34 years, who has been in domestic service, concealing her dread secret until a few weeks ago, when a doctor called upon us, asking for our help. A devoted sister is the other occupant of her small room, which is in nice order, ready for the nurse – a little table being set aside for her dressings and appliances. The patient is very weak, and the disease increasing so rapidly that constant care and good nourishment will be required. Nurse dresses the wound, changes her linen, and makes her comfortable for the time, while urging her to consent to become a candidate at the approaching election at the Royal Hospital for incurables. Her sister is barely able to support herself, and we lend all the necessary comforts; but they are much attached to each other, and disliked the mention of separation. Eventually they yielded to the advice given them by the doctor and nurse, and she was kindly admitted at the December election.[11]

The fundraisers of St Patrick's Home were, of course, competing with other voluntary organisations, including the hospitals, for the assistance of the same small group of wealthy benefactors. The following story, from the same annual report, highlights the benefits of treating people at home rather than at the well-intentioned, but often unyielding, institutions that were available at the time. It concerns a young married woman in great destitution and covered in bedsores.

> She is suffering from paraplegia, and was in hospital for some time, but fretted so much about her children, she persuaded her husband to bring her home. We had taken her to hospital, and fearing to find us angry when we found she had left it, she did not send for us. Nurse was told of her state by another patient, who is a great sufferer from that most dreadful disease, Jacob's ulcer. Her bedsores are now healed, and, to Nurse's great joy, there is a decided improvement in her general condition: real nursing is here required which occupies some time.[12]

Miss Mary Quain described the routine visit she paid to an elderly lady in 1955.

> So she is off again over the hill and dale to Granny Cummins. She is really very well except that she is very old and confined to bed. She needs general attention. Sometimes she can be very difficult but she always welcomes the Nurse. As she approaches, the nurse wonders what will be happening today. Yesterday Granny was very busy fighting the battle of Clontarf and to judge by her general attitude it was just as well for Turgesius that he was not present. Today she is quiet otherwise very well. She is rewarding patient to care for as she looks so clean and tidy after her bath, and appreciates the attention given by the nurse.[13]

In 1959 Miss Sheila Pim, who was a committee member of Dundrum DNA, wrote an article about the daily work of a Jubilee nurse. In the intervening time since 1896 very little in their work practice had changed. 'One patient has to be given an enema, and a bedridden old woman waits anxiously every morning for nurse to come and tidy her up for the day.'[14]

While the service provided by the nurse was free to those who could not afford to pay, a voluntary contribution was expected from those who could. The small brown envelopes were a way of providing discretion to the donors.

> So she puts some collecting envelopes in her bag, and leaves one with a patient who but for her would have to waste hours in an out-patients department waiting to get an injection. The patient puts half a crown in it. Another woman, whose ulcerated leg Nurse has been calling on regularly to dress, puts the envelope on the mantelpiece to wait for her husband's pay day.[15]

The Poultice

In the early stages of the scheme, some form of poultice was used for nearly every ailment. A mustard and linseed poultice could be applied to the chest for bronchitis and pneumonia and a different potion applied to wounds, infections and bed sores. Tepid sponging with a damp cloth to reduce temperatures was also a form of poultice. Replacement and renewal of these balms was done daily but, more often, twice daily. In the absence of antibiotics they offered a palliative comfort, and their renewal offered an opportunity to assess the patient's own healing power.

In 1896 the Annual Report for St Patrick's Home included 'one day's work – a round with a nurse'. Starting from the home at 8.15 in the morning the first visit was to a little boy of two years in a critical state suffering from broncho-pneumonia.

> He has had a restless night – breathing very distressed – but has taken a fair amount of nourishment. Nurse charts the temperature, pulse, and respiration – all very high – and rapidly prepares to give him a refreshing sponging, and to renew his jacket poultices. This is done beside the fire inside a screen made of chairs, with a blanket thrown over them. She then gives him a little wine whey, as ordered, and replaces him in his cradle, adjusting the steam kettle which is kept going night and day, and has the satisfaction of seeing him in a quiet sleep by the time she has written her report for the doctor.[16]

The application of a poultice also provided the nurse with an opportunity for the patient's family to contribute towards the healing process. This was essential in a busy district, and particularly in the case of inaccessible homes, as the nurse was not capable of getting everywhere. In 1904 the Lady Dudley's nurse described this to her committee.

> A child with double pneumonia, to which I was called on Christmas Day. She lived three miles out with no road going to within half a mile of the house. To get there, one had to walk through a swamp for part of the way, and then climb up the mountain side to the house, which was most difficult in this wet and stormy weather, and it was just as difficult to teach the mother of the child how to make a poultice, put it on and keep the child clean. I visited the child twice every day for ten days. She is now convalescent.[17]

In 1908, the doctor had prescribed a poultice but the great advantage for a district with a Queen's nurse was that she showed the people how to apply it, and many other prescriptions, correctly.

> The first patient I had the day after my arrival was a very bad case of pneumonia. Doctor had been with her only once, and left directions that she was to be poulticed, when he was then obliged to leave, just a few days before my arrival. It was just as well for the poor woman that I had arrived in good time. Her people had burned her chest with the poulticing, but not relieved the pain. Patient is now doing very well. She lived five miles from me, and the passage leading to the house was very rough and troublesome to climb.[18]

In 1911 the nurse described a challenging poultice treatment in the west of Ireland.

> My first case was rather a shock to me. Half the room was little more than a dung heap: at the other side was a big turf fire pouring smoke into the room (for there was no chimney), and round it were a man, a woman, five children, a dog, a pig, a cow, a calf, a donkey and four or five fowls. My patient is the baby, very ill with pneumonia, being poulticed twice a day – bran being used in default of linseed. It is the funniest sight in the world to see the whole ragged little family holding out various bits of rag and clothing to the fire to dry and warm preparatory to baby's fresh poultice, and occasionally boxing the pig's ears when he comes too close. I have to do everything on the floor – one piece of paper spread for myself and another for my appliances. But this is all probably quite familiar to you though strange enough to me. The newspaper which came the other day was quite a godsend, not merely for its news but also for its usefulness when read.[19]

POLITICS AND FAMINE

Political and economic conditions in Ireland impacted very directly on the nurses and their patients. The nurses of St Laurence's Home in the north inner city of Dublin found themselves in the very eye of the storm during the 1916 rebellion. Their remit was to treat everybody who needed care regardless of politics or religion. A nurse reporting in the *Queen's Nurses' Magazine* in July 1916 described the effects of the rebellion from the perspective of the nurses who witnessed it.

During Easter week the nurses at St Laurence's Home, Dublin, had many opportunities of showing how well-trained and disciplined nurses could, besides attending on the wounded, help by their calmness to infuse courage into the terror-stricken people. During all those terrible days the Matron and nurses of this Home went about attending to the wounded and comforting the people.

One of the nurses passing a house where a poor woman had been shot through the head was called in and did all possible to maintain life, but the nature of the wound was so terrible that the woman only lived a short time. Nurse stayed until the end, and then rendered the last services.

Many injured persons came to the Home to be dressed, and one nurse remained. On duty there whilst through those days incessant calls were made on the other nurses to go to different part of the city. This work brought them to the most dangerous parts, and where loss of life was greatest, but needless to say they went without the slightest hesitation. The Home is not far from North King Street, so they were of special help in that part where, under ordinary circumstances, their work so often leads them but which now presents a sad and very different aspect.[20]

In 1922, when Ireland was once again embroiled in political turmoil, the economic hardship suffered by the ordinary people was horrendous. It was deeply distressing for the nurses trying to assist with limited means but empathetic hearts. A letter to the *Queen's Nurses' Magazine* from the west of Ireland described the reality of their work under such circumstances.

You must have seen by the papers the deplorable conditions of the poor people in my district. There are hundreds who are absolutely starving, and insufficiently clothed. I have seen families with nothing in the house but a few potatoes, which they boiled and ate during the day; no milk, tea or flour, or means of getting it. Others have nothing but flour which they got from the White Cross Fund. I had a maternity case yesterday where the husband of the patient was an epileptic, and of course had not earned anything for a long time. There were three other children half naked and starving, they had no potatoes, had nothing but black tea and awful bread made of water. The mother lay on a heap of straw at the fireside, and had only a piece of a blanket and a shawl to cover her. These were the only bedclothes they had for the whole family, and of course she had nothing whatever for the new baby. When she wanted a drink I had to give her tea without milk or sugar. I was far away from a shop, and her neighbours were just like herself, none of them were any better off. This is only one of the many examples I meet day after day. There is no employment for those who could work in this particular part. Other families who had cattle to dispose of were badly handicapped as there were no markets for them, and as they were unable to feed them, had let them go for almost nothing to any buyer who came along.

Out of the one hundred and fifty families about one hundred are in the most awful distress. My attention was at first drawn to it by the fact that children were seen in January turning over the soil that was dug last year, searching for stray potatoes. When I had an opportunity to see the mother I found that there was not a morsel of food in the house, the children were so naked that they were hidden away at the approach of a stranger, and only one child of the ten had any clothes to go to school (they were the present of his godparents). One day the teacher was reading to the school of the dreadful suffering in Central Europe, and one of the children said when he came home, 'There was no word of me being hungry, mother!' He had not tasted food from twelve o'clock the previous day. Now that is a type of the suffering. At the meeting which I had already mentioned to you I made the remark that things could hardly be worse than human beings trying to exist on Indian meal porridge taken with a little sugar, and our best helper said, 'are you aware that they have not enough even of that?' A prominent shopkeeper told me last night that many families do not come to the shop any more even for small things; there is no money to pay for them. The chief causes of the distress are the failure of the Donegal Home Spun (large quantities of it lie on the hands of those unfortunate people unsold) and of the embroidery through the boycott of Belfast, as well as the fishing, which failed for the last few seasons, and last, but not least, the failure of the potato crop in 1920, so that no seed was available for 1921, except what the parish priests gave.[21]

TUBERCULOSIS

The sad statistics of 'the white plague' indicate the vast numbers of young people that were taken by tuberculosis. Dying of TB was a gruesome feat in the days before antibiotics and proper analgesics. In 1892, while doing a round with Nurse Ryan in south inner-city Dublin, the reporter for the *Lady of the House* newspaper described the first case visited that day.

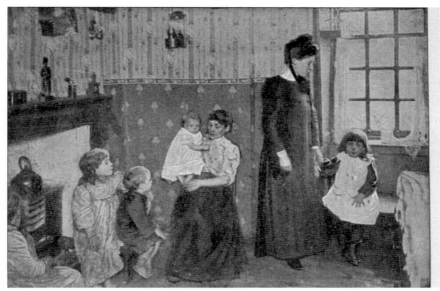

FIRST VISIT OF CONSUMPTION DISPENSARY NURSE TO AN INFECTED HOME.
Courtesy of the National Library of Ireland.

It was that of a young girl in the very last stage of consumption. I had been warned that we might find her dead, and certainly, though still a sentient being, no Egyptian skeleton at the feast could be a more lasting memento mori than that sweet-faced girl with eyes of the Irish grey. For her, clean sheets and a night dress were provided, and little squares of old linen for that fearful expectoration consequent upon her coughing up her lungs; some egg and milk was administered before sad toilet began, and beef tea set on the fire to heat restorative at its close; then the wasted face and poor worn hands were bathed in warm water with a large tangle of soft wood wool, the mouth cleansed and the parched lips moistened with some cooling drops; the body, too, was washed and lightly rubbed over with some protective spirit, and parts where skin appeared in danger of actually being cut through by the bone were anointed and dusted with violet powder; we left the poor patient much fresher, and turned on one side to go to sleep after the exertion of even being made more comfortable.[22]

In the earlier years, great ignorance and fear surrounded the disease, which seemed to encounter no social obstacle and infected every-one. Patients of the tuberculosis Queen's nurse were described in the *Queen's Nurses' Magazine* in December 1908. This nurse had a district of half of Dublin city, either north or south. Patients seen in any of the hospitals were recommended to the nurse for treatment. If they accepted they were visited by her with an everyday programme of care organised for them. This involved the reduction of contamination with the rest of the family, healthy nutrition and fresh air as the main defences against the disease available at the time. Her descriptions feature every member of the family as they were, as was the case with all Jubilee nurses, included in her remit of care.

> One man had been a bottle-blower, he had a wife and seven children who were almost starving as he had been unable to work for two years. They were given food and clothing, money was collected to send him to Newcastle Sanatorium. While he was away the rent was paid, and milk was allowed to the children. When he returned other work was found for him, as it was not considered safe for him to return to his own trade.
>
> Another patient, a boy, was found lying on a mattress on the floor. All the windows were tightly closed, and the family were in a fearful state of poverty. There was a small room which just held a bed. It had a fine large window, but was full of rubbish. It was cleared out, the window-sashes removed, and a bed fixed up in it for the patient, who was also supplied with proper nourishment. He soon improved, then light work was found for him. He has now been working for three months and has not missed one day.[23]

Finally the nurse described the cases of two mothers with TB.

> One woman had a small baby. She could get very little fresh air, as she could not leave the baby, and could not carry it when she went out. She was given a perambulator, and is now out all day. Both mother and baby are much improved. Another woman who was far advanced in tuberculosis was sleeping in the same bed with several small children. She was quite willing to go to hospital, but could not leave the two youngest children. Money was collected and they were boarded out for ten weeks, which enabled her to go to the South Dublin Union.[24]

In the west of Ireland the Lady Dudley's nurse was also dealing with this horrible scourge. Phthisis is another name for TB and in 1908 it was very often fatal.

Got a patient, a young woman of 32 in a very advanced stage of phthisis, sadly neglected with no one to look after her, they were very poor. Visited her every second day, though she was outside District I had to walk 3 miles through a bog. Cleaned her room, made her bed & co dressed bed sores, which were very bad, got her to use sputum cup and disinfectants, kept the young children from her room. She died last week. Her husband cleaned out the house, burning old clothes & c., whitewashed the place, and I gave him some disinfectants to put in the whitewash. Both patient and husband were very grateful for services.[25]

In 1935 there was still an uphill battle against superstition with regard to TB and its treatment. Nurse Clancy in Fanad district in County Donegal was interviewed by the *Nursing Mirror and Midwives Journal* in her new district. The piece described

... a tuberculosis boy. His disease had reached an advanced stage, and Nurse Clancy had been visiting him daily. On one occasion she was confronted at the door of the cottage, and told she need not come any more. The parents had consulted a 'doctor', who had brought a charm from him which the little patient wore round his neck, and no amount of persuasion would shake their faith in their purchase.[26]

Epidemics

Epidemics were terrifying events for medical professionals in the community. When it was possible to keep things under control, as some of these examples show, relief must have been overwhelming. Without antibiotics, antivirals or any other modern treatments there was little that could be done without a village-wide campaign of isolation.

In 1905 the annual report noted that the new Lady Dudley's nurse in Geesala, County Mayo had to cope with both a serious epidemic of measles and an outbreak of typhus in the winter and early spring of that year.

The first Lady Dudley's annual report discussed their taking over the district of Achill Island.

On February 1st Nurse McWilliam was sent to Achill Island. For some years past a Nurse has been maintained in this locality by means of a special fund raised and administered by Queen Victoria's Jubilee Institute. At the request of the Institute in November, 1903, the

Committee took over the control of this district and appointed Nurse McWilliam under the Scheme. She had to begin her duties under somewhat difficult circumstances, owing to a severe epidemic of smallpox which was raging on the Island. She immediately found her hands full and in spite of all drawbacks writes cheerfully and hopefully of her work.[27]

A letter following this from the rector on the island described how happy they were to have the nurse. He also described that there may be resistance from the community but 'The great point is to gain their confidence by a few successful cases and then she will very seldom be idle'.[28]

The eighth annual report in 1910 featured the following:

We had a case of typhoid in the district. This patient has not been well for four weeks though he has been up and tried to do his work, till he was suddenly taken ill with a severe colic, when he was immediately attended to by doctor and myself, and was soon relieved by frequent application of hot turpentine stupes. He has since remained in bed and showed every symptom of typhoid fever, but the attack was a very slight one fortunately. Everything has been done to prevent the spread of the disease so far but we only hope he has not already contaminated any of the neighbouring dwellings.[29]

The same year a letter from a Lady Dudley's nurse described the distress among the medics regarding the resistance of the people to hospital admission.

One typhoid case which was removed to hospital, and which I accidently [sic] discovered on hearing of the boy being ill, and went to see him and discovered his temperature 104', pulse 120. He had also chest crepitation's [sic], but from the parent's statement, I suspected typhoid, and had the doctor sent for. He confirmed my suspicions, but although he had the hospital van sent for patient, the friends would not have him removed. I then got the parish priest to interfere and he insisted on having the patient removed, but it was not until the doctor had to get a magistrate's order the boy was transferred to hospital. He is now progressing very well. The hospital doctors said they never saw such a bad case and only for he being sent in so soon he never would have got better.[30]

INFANTS

One of the primary reasons for setting up the domiciliary nursing scheme was to provide competent, qualified maternity care for women in their own homes. As with all change it was difficult to replace the established 'handy women' in a district. A recurring problem for the pioneer Queen's nurses was this loyalty to the old

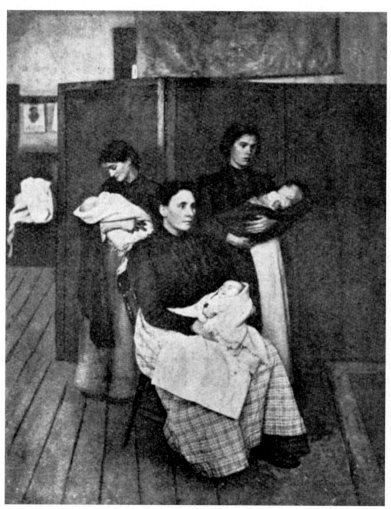

A class during a Baby Club meeting in Blackrock, Co. Cork, 1909. Founded by the WNHA, 'Baby Clubs' assisted young mothers with advice, encouragement and often nourishment in the early part of the twentieth century when there was no other support. Courtesy of the National Library of Ireland.

regime. In 1908 the nurse in a Lady Dudley's district wrote to show how determined she had to be to win over this resistance.

> Maternity – Distance from Nurse's house 8 miles. Call came about 10 p.m. When I got about 2 miles of patient's house we could take the car no further. I was just starting to walk across the mountain when I was met by a party of the patient's friends, who came as the woman was all right, and the night was so dark and raining sleet and show, and the wind blowing in our faces, to try and persuade me not to venture as I could never get there; still I persisted in going. I'm sure it took me a full 2 hours to walk. When I got to the house there was great indignation on the part of the old handy woman, who informed me the patient never had a nurse or doctor for six of a family.[31]

Why she felt this urgency to visit the patient is shown in the next case study, which occurred much earlier and in a completely different district but offers an example of what the early Lady Dudley's nurses could encounter on any call.

> A maternity case and a particularly sad one. The woman lived three miles from the village and this was her eleventh child, and though she had been ill all night it was only at 12.15 p.m. next day that her little girl came for me, with no more urgent message than that her mother was ill. I went at once and on my arrival at the house found the patient practically dying. I immediately sent for the doctor and clergyman though I feared that neither would reach her in time. And in the meantime I did my best for the poor thing, who never rallied but died in about 20 minutes after my arrival. I asked the woman who was with her why she had not sent for assistance sooner, and the excuse given me was that the patient never needed a doctor or a nurse on such occasions, and that she did not think she would need them this time, the woman taking great credit to herself for having sent for me even then. The house was the most wretched one, with practically nothing in it. The patient was lying on a bit of grass on the floor, with no covering except an old skirt and jacket she had on. There was no underclothing, bed or bed-clothing. I could not even get a bit of candle to enable me to see her when I went in. It was the most pitiable state of affairs that anyone could imagine and I shall not forget my experience of that day for some time. A collection is being made in the parish to get some clothes etc. for the children.[32]

The sheer physical strength required for the work of a Queen's nurse is hard to imagine without listening to their own accounts. In 1906 a Lady Dudley nurse wrote of the challenge she faced one winter even before she arrived at her patient's bedside.

> This has been a very heavy month. The midwifery calls came nearly all one after another. I was on duty without sleep or returning home for early 52 hours, all the Christmas in fact. The condition of the roads made it much more hard, as in some places the snow was four feet deep which made it impossible to take a car or ride a bicycle, and you had to struggle through as best you could. However, I am glad to say all the cases have done well and I feel very fit myself to begin another year's work.[33]

An important part of the Jubilee maternity service were the follow-up calls to ensure mother and baby were doing well. Mary Quain describes, in 1955, in note-like language 'A Day in the Life of a Jubilee Nurse'.

> Mrs O'Brien and her new baby are both well. The baby is five days old. Routine care given. The family are well although they are poor. The other children are very pleased with their new sister although the boys think another prospective footballer may have been better. Granny is in charge and Grand-dad keeping an eye on the toddlers. He has a grand way with children and can keep them happy for hours.[34]

Miss Sheila Pim, in an article subtitled 'A District Nurse's Day', concludes her piece in the newspaper of 1959 with a note on the never-ending work day for Queen's nurses.

> As she settles down after tea to write up her files, the telephone rings. Mrs Ryan's baby is not waiting until Sunday. Nurse gets out her scooter again, making sure the lamp is working.[35]

NOTES

1   *Queen's Nurses' Magazine* (May 1904) p. 67, The Queen's Nursing Institute, London.

2   Ibid.

3   B.N. Hedderman, *Glimpses of My Life in Arran* (Bristol: John Wright and Sons, 1917), pp. 82–3.

4   Lady Dudley's Scheme, Annual Report, 1908, p. 15. National Library, Dublin.

5   'In Wildest Donegal: The District Nurses at Fanad Head', *The Nursing Mirror and Midwives Journal* (12 October 1935), p. 27.

6   Lady Dudley's Scheme, Annual Report, 1905/6, p. 13. National Library, Dublin.

7   Lady Dudley's Scheme, Annual Report, 1911, p. 18.

8   *Queen's Nurses' Magazine* (May 1904), p. 12, The Queen's Nursing Institute, London.

9   Lady Dudley's Scheme, Annual Report, 1905/6, p. 19. National Library, Dublin.

10   Lady Dudley's Scheme, Annual Report, 1908, p. 15.

11   St Patrick's Home, Annual Report, 1896, p. 10. National Archives, Dublin.

12   Ibid., p. 9.

13   Mary Quain, 'A Day in the Life of a Jubilee Nurse', *Irish Nursing News* (December/January 1955), p. 6.

14   Sheila Pim, 'A District Nurse's Day: Work, Work, Work', *Irish Times*, Friday 6 November 1955, p. 8. Irish Times Archives.

15   Ibid.

16   St Patrick's Home, Annual Report, 1896, p. 9. National Archives, Dublin.

17   Lady Dudley's Scheme, Annual Report, 1904, p. 14. National Library, Dublin.

18   Lady Dudley's Scheme, Annual Report, 1908, p. 14.

19   Lady Dudley's Scheme, Annual Report, 1911, pp. 16–17.

20   *Queen's Nurses' Magazine* (May 1916), pp. 83–4. The Queen's Nursing Institute, London.

21   *Queen's Nurses' Magazine* (1922), pp. 43–4.

22   Etta Catterson Smith, 'A Day in the Life of a Jubilee Nurse', *The Lady of the House*, 14 April 1892, p. 23. National Library, Dublin.

23   *Queen's Nurses' Magazine* (December 1908), p. 110. The Queen's Nursing Institute, London.

24   Ibid.

25   Lady Dudley's Scheme, 6th Annual Report, 1908, p. 14. National Library, Dublin.

26   'In Wildest Donegal: The District Nurses at Fanad Head'.

27   Lady Dudley's Scheme, 1st Annual Report, 1904, p. 14. National Library, Dublin.

28   Ibid.

29   Lady Dudley's Scheme, Annual Report, 1910, p. 15.

30   Ibid., p. 16.

31   Lady Dudley's Scheme, Annual Report, 1908, p. 15.

32   Lady Dudley's Scheme, Annual Report, 1904/5, p. 14.

33   Lady Dudley's Scheme, Annual Report, 1906, p. 19.

34   Quain, 'A Day in the life of a Jubilee Nurse', p. 6.

35   Pim 'A District Nurse's Day: Work, Work, Work'.

Select Bibliography

PRIMARY SOURCES

The Queen's Nursing Institute, London
Queen's Institute for District Nursing in Ireland, North Brunswick Street, Dublin 7
Wellcome Library, London
University College Dublin, An Bord Altranais, Archives of the Queen's Institute in Ireland

- Jubilee Nurses Affiliated Branches 1890–1967, P220/28–30
- The Roll of Jubilee Nurses 1893–1967, P220/31–7

OPW/NUI Maynooth Archive and Research Centre, Castletown House, Celbridge, County Kildare
The Overend Family Archive, Airfield, Dundrum, Reference number PP/AIR
Donegal County Archives, Lifford, County Donegal, Boxes P27/10 and P48/1–3

- Annual Reports of the County Medical Officer, Donegal

Tipperary County Archives, Clonmel, County Tipperary
Department of Health Archives, Hawkins House, Hawkins Street, Dublin 2
Dublin Diocesan Archives, Archbishop's Palace, Drumcondra, Dublin 9

- Archbishop Walsh Papers, 1890s

The National Library of Ireland, Kildare Street, Dublin 2

- Lady Dudley's Annual Reports
- Pamphlets Collection
- The Journal of The Statistical and Social Inquiry Society of Ireland, 1863

The National Archives of Ireland, Bishop Street, Dublin 8

- Queen's Institute Annual Reports, 1924–1947
- St Patrick's Home Annual Reports, 1889–1905
- Lady Dudley's Annual Reports, Minutes of Monthly Meetings and Photograph Album
- Department of Health Files
- Peamount Archives

NEWSPAPERS AND PERIODICALS

Irish Times
Kildare Observer, 1880–1935
The Lady of the House
Journal of the Statistical and Social Inquiry Society
Irish Nursing News
Nursing Mirror and Midwives Journal
Irish Homestead, Journal of the Agricultural Cooperative Movement
British Medical Journal
New York Times

LETTERS AND MANUSCRIPTS

Birr Castle Archives. This private collection does not have public access. Contact may be possible through the friends of Birr Castle.

Mary Quain's Notes, c/o Ms Therese Meehan, History of Nursing Department, University College Dublin

Mary Quain, address given at the centenary of the Queen's Institute in Belfast, 27 November 1987, Queen's Institute Ireland

Jean Cochrane, Belfast, letter to the authors, 30 May 2011

Mary Duffy, Newtoncunningham, County Donegal, short unpublished memoir

James Muldowney, Professor, Canada, email letter, 31 May 2011

Peter Griffin, Dooneen, County Waterford, email letter, 31 May 2011

BOOKS, ARTICLES AND OTHER PUBLISHED MATERIAL

Barrington, Ruth, *Health Medicine and Politics in Ireland* (Dublin: Institute of Public Administration, 1987)

Catalogue for the Irish International Exhibition 1907, with foreword by the Countess of Aberdeen and a chapter contributed by Lady Dudley

Damant, Margaret, 'A Biographical Profile of Queen's Nurses in Britain 1910–1968', *The Social History of Medicine*, vol. 23, no. 3 (December 2010), pp. 586–601

Fingall, Elizabeth, Countess, *Seventy Years Young* (Dublin: The Lilliput Press, 1991)

Fitzgerald, W.G. (ed.), *The Voice of Ireland* (Dublin: John Heywood Ltd, 1924)

Hedderman, B.N. *Glimpses of My Life in Aran: Some Experiences of a District Nurse in these Remote Islands Off the West Coast of Ireland* (Bristol: John Wright & Sons Ltd, 1917)

Hensey, Brendan, *The Health Services of Ireland* (Dublin: Institute of Public Administration, 1972)

Howse, Carrie, 'The Development of District Nursing in England 1880–1925', *Nursing
History Review* (2007), pp. 65–94

Keane, Maureen, *Ishbel: Lady Aberdeen in Ireland* (Newtownards: Colourpoint Books, 1999)

Meehan, Therese, 'Heading into the Wind: A Jubilee-Dudley Nurse Midwife in West Galway from 1937–1943', in Gerard M. Fealy (ed.), *Care to Remember: Nursing and Midwifery in Ireland* (Cork: Mercier Press, 2005)

Micks, William L. *The Congested Districts Board for Ireland 1891–1923* (Dublin: Eason & Son Ltd, 1925)

Murray, James P. *Galway: A Medico-Social History* (Galway: Kenny's Bookshop, 1994)

Nightingale, Florence, *On Trained Nursing for the Sick Poor* (pamphlet) (London: Archives of Queen's Nurse Institute, 1881)

O'Brien, Sophie, 'The Mallow Jubilee Nurse', in *My Irish Friends* (Dublin and London: Burns, Oates & Washbourne, 1937)

Ó Cléirigh, Nellie, *Hardship and High Living: Irish Women's Lives 1808–1923* (Dublin: Portobello Press, 2003)

Ó hÓgartaigh, Margaret, *Quiet Revolutionaries: Irish Women in Education, Medicine and Sport, 1861–1964* (Dublin: The History Press Ireland, 2011)

Queen's Nursing Institute, *QNI 125*, privately published book on the history of the Queen's Institute to celebrate its 125th anniversary, 2012

Rathbone, William, 'Introduction', in *The History and Progress of District Nursing* (London: Macmillan, 1890)

Smithson, Annie M.P. *Her Irish Heritage* (Dublin: Talbot Press, 1918)

Smithson, Annie M.P. *Carmen Cavanagh* (Dublin: Talbot Press, 1921)

Smithson, Annie M.P. *The Marriage of Nurse Harding* (Dublin and Cork: Mercier Press, 1989)

Smithson, Annie M.P. *Myself and Others: An Autobiography* (Dublin: Talbot Press, 1945)

Stocks, Mary, *A Hundred Years of District Nursing* (London: Allen & Unwin, 1960)

Wickham, Ann, 'The Nursing Radicalism of the Honourable Albina Broderick 1861–1955',

Nursing History Review, vol. 15 (2007), pp. 51–64

INTERVIEWS

Nurses

Mary Byrne and Phyllis Nelson, Tullamore, County Offaly, 29 April 2010

Jenny Ledingham, Dún Laoghaire, County Dublin, August and September 2010

Bernie Hartery (nee Coleman), Phyllis Fennelly (nee Meally) and Anne Connolly (nee Barry), Waterford, 12 November 2010

Mary Kiernan, Interview with Dr Vincent Pippett, Wicklow, 7 June 2011

Maura Kilmartin, Dundrum, Dublin 14, July, August and October 2011

Mary Duffy and daughter Delia, Newtowncunningham, County Donegal, 27 September 2011

Rita Pearson, Johnstown, County Donegal, 27 October 2011

District Nursing Associations

Portmarnock: Maura Kennedy, Malahide, 24 September 2009

Ballinasloe, County Galway: Rory Kilduff and Matthew Ganly, 6 August 2010

Lady Dudley's Scheme Administration: Sheila McCrann, 14 March 2012

Birr, County Offaly: Kathleen McEvoy, Rathmines, Dublin 6, 10 June 2011

Dalkey and Ballybrack: Joan Hall and Anne Purcell, Sandycove, County Dublin, 20 July 2011

Newtowncunningham, County Donegal: Group Interview in the Home of Michael and Kate Chance, Manorcunningham, County Donegal, 11 August 2011

Mountcharles, County Donegal: Mary Nolan, 12 August 2011

Cavan: Dr Áine Sullivan, 6 September 2011

APPENDIX 1

Districts Affiliated with the Queen's Institute of Ireland

Page No.	District	Scheme	Opened	Nurses	Closed	Longstanding Individual Nurses
553 v2*	Achill Sound, Co. Mayo	LDS**	1918	2	1925	
235	Achill, Co. Mayo	LDS	1897	24	1967	
91–337 v3	Adare, Co. Limerick	DNA	1931	8	1966	Mary Elizabeth O'Loughlin 1941–1958
73 v3	Adrigole, Co. Cork	LDS	1929	1	1934	
213–14 v3	Adrigole, Co. Cork (Part 2)	DNA	1936	8	1962	
13–15 v2	Aghir, Enfield, Co. Meath	DNA	1907	16	1961	Susan Weldon 1912–1930

* Page numbers refer to the original three volumes of the Queen's Institute records of district nursing associations affiliated. The first volume is just numbered, the second volume is denoted as v2 and the third volume as v3.

** LDS: Lady Dudley's Scheme

DNA: District Nursing Association

WNHA: Women's National Health Association

Home: Care facilities where individuals, particularly children, were sent for rest. The exceptions were St Laurence's and St Patrick's Homes, which were training and residential facilities for Queen's nurses.

Page No.	District	Scheme	Opened	Nurses	Closed	Longstanding Individual Nurses
547–50	Anagry, Co. Donegal	LDS	1905	17	1966	
161–2 v3	Annamoe, Co. Wicklow	DNA	1933	7	1958	
217	Antrim & Muckamore, Co. Antrim	DNA	1897	1	1929	Annie Fleming 1897–1933
143–369 v3	Ardara, Co. Donegal	LDS	1932	9	1967	Mary Josephine Scanlon 1950–1967
481–4	Ardee, Co. Louth	DNA	1903	19	1964	
379–80	Ardmore, Co. Waterford	DNA	1901	5	1922	
275–6 v3	Ardmore/Grange, Co. Waterford (Part 2)	DNA	1943	6	1966	
373 v2	Ardstraw, Co. Tyrone	DNA	1912	2	1915	
385–8	Arklow, Co. Wicklow	DNA	1901	20	1966	Bridget Byrne nee Jones 1930–1964
301–2	Armagh, Co. Armagh	DNA	1897	19	1929	
505–7	Arranmore Island, Co. Donegal	LDS	1904	19	1966	Elizabeth Scully 1916–1945
583 v2	Athboy, Co. Meath	DNA	1919	1	1929	
529–31 v2	Athlone, Co. Westmeath	DNA	1918	15	1966	Katherine Marinan 1922–1949
253 v2	Athy, Co. Kildare	WNHA	1909	1	1913	
219–20 v3	Athy, Co. Kildare (Part 2)	DNA	1937	8	1966	Theresa Brennan 1950–1966
103	Aughrim, Co. Wicklow	DNA	1894	3	1917	
43 v3	Bagnalstown, Co. Carlow	DNA	1925	3	1934	

Page No.	District	Scheme	Opened	Nurses	Closed	Longstanding Individual Nurses
255–6 v3	Bagnalstown, Co. Carlow (Part 2)	DNA	1942	6	1966	
241–2 v3	Balbriggan, Co. Dublin	DNA	1940	5	1956	
541 v2	Ballaghadereen, Co. Roscommon	LDS/DNA	1919	3	1925	
499	Ballina & Killaloe, Co. Tipperary	DNA	1903	6	1920	
307 v2	Ballina, Co. Mayo	DNA	1912	4	1920	
93–4 v3	Ballina, Co. Mayo	DNA	1931	1	1958	Mary Jane Durr 1931–1958
225 v3	Ballinafad, Co. Roscommon	LDS	1938	3	1945	
451 v2	Ballinakill, Queen's County (Now Co. Laois)	DNA	1917	2	1919	
181 v2	Ballinalea, Edgwardstown & Granard, Co. Longford	WNHA	1909	3	1913	
265	Ballinamallard, Co. Fermanagh	DNA	1898	3	1903	
127 v2	Ballinasloe, Co. Galway	WNHA	1908	1	1911	
209–10 v3	Ballinasloe, Co. Galway (Part 2)	DNA	1936	1	1955	Mary Agnes O'Grady 1936–1955
77 v3	Ballycarry & Islandmagee, Co. Antrim	DNA	1929	1	1929	
109	Ballycastle, Co. Antrim	DNA	1894	5	1929	Mary F. Hipwell 1900–1921
133–4 v3	Ballyconnelly, Co. Galway	LDS	1932	8	1959	

Page No.	District	Scheme	Opened	Nurses	Closed	Longstanding Individual Nurses
439–40	Ballycroy, Co. Mayo	LDS	1903	3	1912	
97–8 v3	Ballycroy, Co. Mayo	LDS	1931	5	1945	
535	Ballyduff, Co. Kerry	DNA	1904	1	1909	
201–2 v3	Ballyferriter, Co. Kerry	DNA	1935	5	1962	
263 v3	Ballyglas, Co. Galway	DNA	1943	3	1954	
535–7 v2	Ballyhaunis, Co. Mayo	LDS	1919	7	1967	Theresa Whitside 1919–1938; Lena Kelly 1945–1956
35 v3	Ballykinlar, Camp, Co. Down	DNA	1924	1	1925	
203–4 v3	Ballymacaward & Woodlawn, Co. Galway	DNA	1935	9	1951	
31–3	Ballymena, Co. Antrim	DNA	1881	18	1929	
553–4	Ballymoney, Co. Antrim	DNA	1905	3	1929	
109 v3	Ballyragget & Castlecomer, Co. Kilkenny	DNA	1931	15	1964	
133–5 v2	Ballyshannon, Co. Donegal	WNHA	1909	9	1967	Catherine Hart 1909–1941
115	Banbridge, Co. Down	DNA	1894	11	1929	Lizzi Jane Browne 1910–1941
223	Bangor, Co. Down	DNA	1897	24	1929	
463–6	Bealadangan, Co. Galway	LDS	1903	30	1967	
235 v2	Beleek, Co. Fermanagh	WNHA	1910	2	1922	
421–2 v2	Beleek, Co. Fermanagh (Part 2)	DNA	1914	4	1930	

Page No.	District	Scheme	Opened	Nurses	Closed	Longstanding Individual Nurses
43 v2	Belfast, Co. Antrim	WNHA	1908	3	1913	
95–355 v3	Bennetsbridge, Co. Kilkenny	DNA	1931	12	1966	
559–62	Birr, Kings County (Now Co. Offaly)	DNA	1906	12	1966	
241	Blackrock, Booterstown & Stillorgan, Co. Dublin	DNA	1896	10	1950	Margaret F. Noblett 1902–1933
81–2 v3	Blacksod, Co. Mayo	LDS	1929	16	1956	
379 v2	Blarney, Co. Cork	DNA	1912	7	1921	
211–12 v3	Blessington, Co. Wicklow	DNA	1936	7	1958	
475 v2	Borris, Co. Carlow	DNA	1914	1	1947	
181–2 3v	Borris, Co. Carlow	DNA	1934	7	1947	
247	Bray, Co. Wicklow	WNHA	1908	4	1929	
247 v2	Bray, Co. Wicklow	WNHA	1908	3	1929	
187	Bray, Fr. Healy, Co. Wicklow	DNA	1896	6	1966	Josephine Purcell 1897–1937
67 v3	Bronghshaw, Co. Antrim	DNA	1929	1	1929	
53–4 v3	Bruckless&Dunkineely, Co. Donegal	LDS	1927	14	1958	
205	Buncrana, Co. Donegal	DNA	1896	26	1966	
197–8 v3	Bundoran, Co. Donegal	DNA	1935	2	1962	Kathleen Henry 1940–1962
277	Burriscarra, Co. Mayo	DNA	1898	3	1904	
151	Bushmills, Co. Antrim	DNA	1889	3	1913	

Page No.	District	Scheme	Opened	Nurses	Closed	Longstanding Individual Nurses
571–4	Caherdaniel, Co. Kerry	LDS	1906	14	1966	Catherine Foley 1938–1966
307–10	Cahir, Co. Tipperary	DNA	1896	16	1966	
221–2 v3	Cape Clear Island, Co. Cork	LDS	1937	22	1963	
241	Cappoquinn, Co. Waterford	DNA	1896	19	1958	
89–90 v3	Carbury, Co. Kildare	DNA	1930	9	1947	
355–7 v2	Carlow, Co. Carlow	WNHA	1909	15	1966	
469–72	Carna, Co. Galway	LDS	1903	31	1967	Mary Carr 1948–1967
99–345 v3	Carndonagh Health Club, Co. Donegal	DNA	1931	7	1967	
117–333 v3	Carraroe, Co. Galway	LDS	1932	14	1966	
295 v3	Carrickbyrne, Co. Wexford	DNA	1947	2	1950	
247	Carrickfergus, Co. Antrim	DNA	1897	12	1929	
185–6 v3	Carrickmacross, Co. Monaghan	DNA	1934	5	1948	
391–2 v2	Carrick–on–Shannon, Co. Leitrim	WNHA	1913	2	1929	
391	Carrick–on–Suir, Co. Tipperary	DNA	1901	9	1922	
113–114 v.3	Carrick–on–Suir, Co. Tipperary (Part 2)	DNA	1931	3	1962	Mary Bridget McMahon 1932–1962
259 v3	Carrigalass, Co. Longford	DNA	1942	1	1948	
159–363 v3	Carrigart, Co. Donegal	LDS	1933	Unclear	1959	

Page No.	District	Scheme	Opened	Nurses	Closed	Longstanding Individual Nurses
49–52 v2	Cashel, Co. Tipperary	DNA	1908	25	1966	
409 v2	Castlebar, Co. Mayo	WNHA	1913	1	1914	
415–18	Castlebellingham, Co. Louth	DNA	1902	16	1966	Josephine Bird 1909–1925; Margaret Murphy 1950–1966
11 v3	Castlecaulfield, Co. Tyrone	DNA	1900	3	1929	
187 v2	Castlecomer, Co. Kilkenny	WNHA	1909	2	1919	
65 v3	Castlegregory, Co. Kerry	DNA	1929	5	1932	
51–331 v3	Castlehaven, Co. Cork	DNA	1926	27	1966	
349–52	Castleknock, Co. Dublin	DNA	1901	5	1966	Camilla Dowling 1906–1929; Mary Doyle 1936–1966
283 v3	Castlerea, Co. Roscommon	DNA	1944	5	1953	
147–8 v3	Castletownberehaven, Co. Cork	DNA	1932	9	1958	
343 v2	Cavan, Co. Cavan	WNHA	1911	1	1913	
293–4 v3	Cavan, Co. Cavan (Part 2)	DNA	1946	7	1967	
211 v2	Celbridge & Straffan, Co. Kildare	WNHA	1910	4	1922	
571–3 v2	Charlestown, Co. Mayo	LDS	1918	11	1957	
127	Charleville, Co. Cork	DNA	1894	4	1910	
583–4	Cheeverstown & Clondalkin, Co. Dublin	Home	1905	10	1927	

Page No.	District	Scheme	Opened	Nurses	Closed	Longstanding Individual Nurses
125–6 v3	Clane, Co. Kildare	DNA	1932	11	1959	
481–3 v2	Clara, King's County (Now Co. Offaly)	DNA	1914	3	1957	Sarah E. McDermott 1914–1951
167–8 v3	Clare Island, Co. Mayo	DNA	1933	12	1950	
451	Clarina, Patrickswell & Roxburgh, Co. Limerick	DNA	1903	4	1907	
69–70 v3	Cleggan, Co. Galway	LDS	1929	14	1966	
259 v2	Clifden, Co. Galway	DNA	1909	1	1914	
273 v3	Clogheen & Ardfinnan, Co. Tipperary	DNA	1943	3	1951	
57–325 v3	Clonbur, Co. Galway	LDS	1928	18	1967	
337–9 v2	Clondalkin, Palmerstown & Chapelizod, Co. Dublin	WNHA	1912	4	1954	Ellen Brophy 1925–1954
229 v2	Clones, Co. Monaghan	WNHA	1909	1	1911	
279–80 v3	Clones, Co. Monaghan	DNA	1944	8	1957	
183–4 v3	Clonmany, Co. Donegal	DNA	1934	6	1959	
427–30	Clonmel, Co. Tipperary	DNA	1903	13	1966	ElizabethMcKillen 1903–1929; Alice Dunne 1930–1947
79–80	Colraine Cottage Hospital, Co. Londonderry	DNA	1893	13	1929	
179–80 v3	Convoy, Co. Donegal	DNA	1934	10	1965	
331 v2	Coole North West, Co. Meath	DNA	1912	1	1920	

Page No.	District	Scheme	Opened	Nurses	Closed	Longstanding Individual Nurses
129 v3	Coole, Co. Westmeath	DNA	1932	2	1935	
85	Coole, Mayne & Kiltoom, Co. Westmeath	DNA	1894	3	1897	
361–4	Cork, Co. Cork	DNA	1900	10	1966	Charlotte Baxter 1905–1931; Ivy Rebecca Keynes 1938–1961
61 v2	Cork, Co. Cork	WNHA	1907	2	1920	
83–4 v3	Cornamona, Co. Galway	LDS	1930	8	1959	
385 v2	Corporation of City of Dublin	WNHA	1906	3	1918	
287–9 v3	Creeslough, Co. Donegal	DNA	1945	5	1967	
433–6 v2	Crosmolina, Co. Mayo	LDS	1914	15	1967	Augusta Mary Norton 1938–1966
343	Crumlin, Co. Antrim	DNA	1901	5	1914	
41 v3	Culmullen & Dunshaughlin, Co. Meath	DNA	1924	10	1956	
55	Curragh Camp, Co. Kildare	DNA	1892	1	1898	
1 v3	Currane & Achill, Co. Mayo	LDS	1919	1	1924	
43	Cushendall Cottage Hospital, Co. Antrim	DNA	1893	6	1903	
49–52	Dalkey, Killiney & Ballybrack, Co. Dublin	DNA	1893	28	1966	Kathleen Blake 1902–1921
493	Dartrey, Co. Monaghan	DNA	1903	2	1907	
257–8 v3	Delvin, Co. Westmeath	DNA	1942	11	1961	

Page No.	District	Scheme	Opened	Nurses	Closed	Longstanding Individual Nurses
37–9 v2	Derrybeg, Co. Donegal	LDS	1908	29	1967	
595–6	Donaraile & Shanballymore, Co. Cork	DNA	1906	4	1921	
131–2 v3	Donegal, Co. Donegal	DNA	1932	6	1962	Mary Fenlon 1934–1956
297 v3	Doneraile & Shanballymore, Co. Cork	DNA	1950	4	1956	
163–4 v3	Doocherry, Co. Donegal	LDS	1933	15	1958	
475–8	Dooks, Co. Kerry	LDS	1903	25	1966	
195–371 v3	Doonamon, Co. Mayo	DNA	1935	11	1966	Kathleen Walsh nee Murphy 1953–1966
319 v3	Downstrands, Co. Donegal	DNA	1956	2	1961	
61–3	Drogheda, Co. Louth	DNA	1893	15	1925	
523–5 v2	Drumholm, Co. Donegal	DNA	1916	Unclear	1966	Dora McVitty nee Black 1918–1954
177–357 v3	Drummin, Co. Mayo	DNA	1934	4	1962	Delia Hoban nee Ward 1941–1962
217 v2	Dublin Branch WNHA	WNHA	1908	8	1914	
415–17 v2	Dunboyne, Clonee, Kilbride, Kilclone, Ballymaglassan, Co. Meath	DNA	1914	13	1967	
139	Dundalk, Co. Louth	DNA	1895	25	1966	M.T. Nolan1944–1966

Page No.	District	Scheme	Opened	Nurses	Closed	Longstanding Individual Nurses
427–9 v2	Dundrum, Sandyford, Milltown & Clonskeagh, Co. Dublin (Part 2)	WNHA	1912	12	1967	
173–4 v3	Dunfanaghy, Co. Donegal	DNA	1933	4	1951	
67–8	Dungannon, Co. Tyrone	DNA	1893	7	1929	
87–8 v3	Dungarvan, Co. Waterford	DNA	1930	7	1956	
127 v3	Dungloe, Co. Donegal	DNA	1932	10	1965	
103–341 v3	Dunmore East, Co. Waterford	DNA	1931	1	1966	Ellen Josephine Barry 1931–1966
277 v2	Dunshaughlin, Co. Meath	DNA	1911	3	1914	
67–8 v2	East Galway, Co. Galway	DNA	1908	6	1925	
505–6 v2	Eglington, Co. Londonderry	DNA	1914	8	1929	
369 v2	Enfield & Longwood, Co. Meath	WNHA	1912	9	1957	Mary Alice Flanagan 1931–1957
47–329 v3	Ennis, Co. Clare	DNA	1908	9	1966	
97	Enniscorthy, Co. Wexford	DNA	1894	4	1909	
193–5 v2	Enniscorthy, Co. Wexford (Part 2)	DNA	1909	4	1961	Grace Hardy 1909–1939; Mary Hennessy 1945–1961
163	Enniskillen, Co. Fermanagh	DNA	1895	11	1929	
169 v3	Fahan/Inch, Co. Donegal	DNA	1933	1	1967	Catherine Reilly 1933–1967
265–7 v2	Fairymount, Co. Roscommon	LDS	1911	12	1967	Mary Ellen McCabe 1936–1960

Page No.	District	Scheme	Opened	Nurses	Closed	Longstanding Individual Nurses
123–361 v3	Fanad, Co. Donegal	DNA	1932	14	1966	
139–40 v3	Fethard, Co. Tipperary	DNA	1932	7	1954	
193–4 v3	Finney, Co. Galway	LDS	1935	5	1955	
565	Foxford, Co. Mayo	LDS	1905	3	1909	
577–9 v2	Foxford, Co. Mayo (Part 2)	DNA	1918	12	1967	Kate Carney 1947–1967
541–4	Foxrock & Stillorgan, Co. Dublin	DNA	1905	13	1966	Annie McKeon 1905–1921; Nora O'Leary 1922–1937
175–375 v3	Freshford, Co. Kilkenny	DNA	1916	15	1966	
155–6 v3	Frosses, Co. Donegal	LDS	1933	9	1966	
59 v3	Galgorm & Cullybackey, Co. Antrim	DNA	1928	1	1929	
259–62	Galway District Nursing Association	DNA	1893	9	1966	Katherine Young 1897–1925; Jane Kelly 1926–1955
237–8 v3	Galway, Co. Galway	DNA	1939	11	1966	
199 v2	Gartan, Co. Donegal	DNA	1909	4	1920	
457–60	Geesala, Co. Mayo	LDS	1903	26	1966	
355–6	Gilford, Co. Down	DNA	1901	9	1929	
107–8 v3	Glangevlin, Co. Cavan	LDS	1931	7	1950	
269 v3	Glasthule, Co. Dublin	DNA	1943	3	1949	
577–80	Glencomcille, Mallinamore & Malinabeg, Co. Donegal	LDS	1906	26	1967	

Page No.	District	Scheme	Opened	Nurses	Closed	Longstanding Individual Nurses
589–92	Glencullen & Sandyford, Co. Dublin	DNA	1906	9	1966	Jennie Jackson 1914–1930; Elizabeth Kathleen Conlisk 1932–1966
9 v3	Glendermott, Co. Londonderry	DNA	1920	4	1926	
247–8 v3	Glenfinn, Co. Donegal	DNA	1940	4	1956	
511–14	Glengarriff, Co. Cork	DNA	1904	15	1966	
19–20 v3	Gortahurk, Co. Donegal	LDS	1920	8	1965	
19–20 v2	Grange Con, Co. Wicklow	DNA	1907	6	1933	
595–7 v2	Greystones & Delgany, Co. Wicklow	DNA	1919	14	1967	
313	Hillsborough, Co. Down	DNA	1899	4	1904	
331–2	Hollywood & Craigavad, Co. Down	DNA	1894	14	1929	
517–18	Hospital & Knocklong, Co. Limerick	DNA	1904	10	1919	
397–400	Howth & Sutton, Co. Dublin	DNA	1902	5	1966	Hannah Roche 1913–1935; Helen Finnegan 1945–1960
187–8 v3	Innishere, Co. Galway	LDS	1934	20	1966	
207 v3	Innismann/Innismore, Co. Galway	LDS	1936	12	1966	
529–32	Inver & Spiddal, Co. Galway	LDS	1904	28	1967	

Page No.	District	Scheme	Opened	Nurses	Closed	Longstanding Individual Nurses
31 v3	Irvinstown, Balllinamallard & Lisnarick, Co. Fermanagh	DNA	1923	3	1929	
267 v3	Kells, Co. Kilkenny	DNA	1943	4	1947	Susan O'Flynn 1915–1935;
31–4 v2	Kells, Co. Meath	DNA	1905	9	1967	Eileen ItaMcGann 1944–1961
367–9	Kenmare, Co. Kerry	DNA	1901	3	1949	
141–358 v3	Kilcar, Co. Donegal	LDS	1932	9	1966	
457–9 v2	Kilcock, Co. Kildare	DNA	1917	10	1967	Mary Elizabeth Quigley 1935–60
373–6	Kilcommin–Erris, Co. Mayo	DNA/LDS	1901	35	1967	
121 v3	Kilcooley, Urlingford & Gortnahoe, Co. Kilkenny	DNA	1932	3	1935	
17–19 v3	Kilcullen, Co. Kildare	DNA	1920	11	1961	Margaret Anne McClean 1928–1954
15–16 v3	Kildare, Co. Kildare	DNA	1920	4	1947	Annie Armstrong 1927–1947
265–7 v3	Kilfinane, Co. Limerick	DNA	1943	5	1967	Imelda O'Hanlon nee Lynch 1943–1967
565–6 v2	Kilkelly, Co. Mayo	LDS	1919	3	1930	
133	Kilkenny, Co. Kilkenny	DNA	1894	22	1958	Anna Parr 1899–1930
227–8 v3	Kilkerrin, Co. Galway	LDS	1938	15	1955	
463–5 v2	Kill, Co. Kildare	DNA	1917	10	1963	Margaret Enright 1932–1949
257 v3	Killane, Co. Waterford	DNA	1941	4	1947	

Page No.	District	Scheme	Opened	Nurses	Closed	Longstanding Individual Nurses
307	Killarney, Co. Kerry	DNA	1899	10	1956	Sophia Murless 1900–1917; Brigid O'Hanlon1927–1947
403–4 v2	Killeshandra, Co. Cavan	WNHA	1913	4	1926	
439 v2	Killorglin & Miltown, Co. Kerry	WNHA	1914	1	1914	
73–6 v2	Killucan & Kinnegad, Co. Westmeath	DNA	1908	5	1966	Kathleen O'Boyle 1927–1966
229–30 v3	Kilmacthomas, Co. Waterford	DNA	1938	5	1947	
27–312 v3	Kilmeaden, Co. Waterford	DNA	1919	15	1966	
25–8 v2	Kiltimagh, Co. Mayo	LDS	1907	20	1967	
63 v3	Lauragh, Co. Kerry	DNA	1928	3	1932	
13 v3	Letterkenny, Co. Donegal	DNA	1919	6	1965	Hanna Sweeney 1929–1965
215–16 v3	Lettermore & Lettermullen, Co. Galway	LDS	1936	16	1964	
153–4 v3	Lifford, Co. Donegal	DNA	1932	8	1958	
25–6	Limavady, Co. Derry	DNA	1890	5	1929	
229	Limerick District Nursing Association, Co. Limerick	DNA	1897	12	1950	
289–91 v2	Lismore, Co. Waterford	DNA	1911	10	1966	Ellen O'Sullivan nee Clifford 1949–1966
361 v2	Lissadell, Co. Sligo	DNA	1912	1	1922	
313–15 v2	Listowel, Co. Kerry	WNHA	1912	4	1966	

Page No.	District	Scheme	Opened	Nurses	Closed	Longstanding Individual Nurses
13–15	Londonderry Nurses' Home	DNA	1891	70	1929	
301–3 v2	Longford, Co. Longford	WNHA	1909	3	1961	Catherine Cunningham nee Greene 1940–1967
319–22 v2	Lucan, Co. Dublin	DNA	1911	29	1967	
2 v3	Malahide, Co. Dublin (Part 2)	DNA	1919	7	1966	
243–4 v3	Malin Head, Co. Donegal	DNA	1940	1	1963	Mary Ellen Collins 1940–1963
121	Mallow, Co. Cork	DNA	1895	12	1962	Emily Gillespie 1901–1922; Bridget Murphy 1939–1962
253–4 v3	Manorcunningham, Co. Donegal	DNA	1941	6	1966	
22 v3	Maryborough, Queen's County (Portlaoise, Co. Laois)	DNA	1916	6	1964	Kathleen Mary O'Leary 1919–1939
55–8 v2	Maynooth, Co. Kildare	DNA	1908	6	1967	Annie McNamara 1922–1946; Gertrude Hyland 1946–1967
103–5 v2	Middleton, Co. Cork	DNA	1908	5	1964	Margaret Jones 1909–1925; Elizabeth O'Keefe nee Nolan 1938–1964
79 v3	Miltown, Tartarafhan & Drumcree, Co. Armagh	DNA	1929	1	1929	
289–90	Miltown, Windyarbour, Clonskeagh & Dundrum, Co. Dublin	DNA	1898	2	1908	
499 v2	Mohill, Co. Leitrim	DNA	1914	4	1920	

Page No.	District	Scheme	Opened	Nurses	Closed	Longstanding Individual Nurses
295–7 v2	Monasterevin, Co. Kildare	WNHA	1909	6	1967	Nellie Horgan 1931–1966; Mary Brick 1947–1966
291–2 v3	Mooncoin, Co. Kilkenny	DNA	1945	4	1956	
403	Mount Talbot, Co. Roscommon	DNA	1901	6	1910	
261–2 v3	Mountmellick, Co. Laois	DNA	1942	2	1964	
55 v3	MountStewart & Greyabbey, Co. Down	DNA	1927	1	1929	
205–6 v3	Moville, Co. Donegal	DNA	1935	2	1963	Mary Elizabeth Tully 1937–1963
5–8 v3	Moycullen, Co. Galway	DNA	1919	16	1967	Mary M. Doherty 1936–1950; Josephine E. Doherty 1936–1960
239–40 v3	Muff & Upper Moville, Co. Donegal	DNA	1939	7	1962	
121–2 v2	Mullingar, Co. Westmeath	DNA	1908	2	1923	
281–2 v3	Mullingar, Co. Westmeath	DNA	1944	2	1966	Julia Loretta O'Dowd 1949–1966
241–2 v2	Mulroy, Co. Donegal	LDS	1910	5	1922	
271–2 v3	Multifarnham & Crookedwood, Co. Westmeath	DNA	1943	5	1962	
145	Naas, Co. Kildare	DNA	1895	28	1967	Cecilia Dillon 1929–1963
139–41 v2	Navan, Co. Meath	WNHA	1909	13	1949	
85–7 v2	Nenagh, Co. Tipperary	DNA	1908	13	1959	Kathleen Ranahan 1929–1945

Page No.	District	Scheme	Opened	Nurses	Closed	Longstanding Individual Nurses
157	Newbridge, Co. Kildare	DNA	1896	9	1964	Una Connolly 1922–1942
409	Newmarket–on–Fergus, Co. Clare	DNA	1902	3	1910	
445–8	Newross, Co. Wexford	DNA	1903	9	1966	Rose Nolan 1907–1923; Rose Lappin 1926–1960
295–6	Newry, Co. Down	DNA	1899	14	1929	
181	Newtownards, Co. Down	DNA	1893	3	1929	Harriet Fleming 1903–1931
1–2 v2	Newtownbarry, Co. Wexford	DNA	1907	9	1919	
7–8 v2	Newtownbreda, Co. Down	DNA	1907	5	1929	
301–2 v3	Newtowncunningham, Co. Donegal	DNA	1950	6	1967	
469–71 v2	Newtownforbes, Co. Longford	DNA	1919	5	1954	Margaret Carbury 1921–1954
137–349 v3	Newtownmountkennedy, Co. Wicklow (Part 2)	DNA	1932	8	1965	
145 v2	Newtownmountkennedy, Newcastle & Kilcock Co. Wicklow	WNHA	1909	2	1912	
19–20	Omagh, Co. Tyrone	DNA	1891	11	1929	
271–2	Ouchterard, Co. Galway	DNA	1898	2	1917	
115–16 v3	Partree, Co. Galway	LDS	1932	9	1956	
283 v2	Pembroke Township, Co. Dublin	WNHA	1911	1	1915	

Page No.	District	Scheme	Opened	Nurses	Closed	Longstanding Individual Nurses
199	Portadown, Co. Armagh	DNA	1887	24	1929	
303–4 v3	Portarlington (Part 2)	DNA	1955	4	1966	
445 v2	Portarlington, Queen's County (Now Co. Laois)	WNHA	1914	5	1921	
39–46 v3	Portlaw, Co. Waterford	DNA	1924	22	1966	
119–20 v3	Portmagee, Co. Kerry	DNA	1932	6	1948	
283–6	Portmarnock, Co. Dublin	DNA	1898	10	1966	
169	Portrush, Co. Antrim	DNA	1895	3	1905	
193	Powerscourt & Kilbride, Co. Wicklow	DNA	1896	15	1966	
151–2 v2	Poyntzpass, Co. Armagh	DNA	1909	6	1923	
151–2 v3	Ramelton, Co. Donegal	DNA	1932	12	1966	
289 v3	Raphoe, Co. Donegal	DNA	1945	2	1950	
321 v3	Raphoe, Co. Donegal (Reorganised)	DNA	1958	3	1967	
75–338 v3	Rathaspeak, Co. Waterford	DNA	1929	2	1962	Theresa Kehoe 1931–1960
277–8 v3	Rathcoole, Co. Dublin	DNA	1944	10	1966	
433–6	Rathfarnham & Whitechurch, Co. Dublin	DNA	1902	10	1966	Mary Anne O'Reilly 1941–1966
163–4 v2	Rathgar & Terenure, Co. Dublin	WNHA	1909	3	1930	Gertrude Sullivan 1917–1932. DNA Amalgamated

Page No.	District	Scheme	Opened	Nurses	Closed	Longstanding Individual Nurses
71–2 v3	Rathlacken, Co. Mayo	LDS	1929	16	1957	
149–50 v3	Rathmullen, Co. Donegal	DNA	1932	5	1967	Winifred Lawless 1951–1967
115–17 v2	Recess, Co. Galway	LDS	1908	19	1959	
165–367 v3	Renvyle & TullyCross, Co. Galway	LDS	1933	11	1967	
33 v3	Resh, Ederney & Lock, Co. Fermanagh	DNA	1923	3	1930	
23–4 v3	Robertstown, Co. Kildare	DNA	1921	13	1950	
487	Roscommon, Co. Roscommon	LDS	1903	2	1906	
49–323 v3	Rosmuck, Co. Galway	LDS	1925	14	1967	
37 v3	Rostrevor, Co. Down	DNA	1924	2	1929	
523–6	Roundstone, Cashel, Co. Galway	LDS	1903	15	1967	
317 v3	Rush & Lusk, Co. Dublin	DNA	1954	2	1962	
29–32 v3	Screen, Co. Sligo	LDS	1921	7	1967	Mary Kelly 1925–1951
231–2 v3	Shankill, Co. Dublin	DNA	1938	1	1966	Mary Ellen Richardson nee Casey 1938–1966
111 v3	Shillelagh & Carnew, Co. Wicklow	DNA	1931	2	1939	
233–4 v3	SieveRua, Co. Kilkenny	DNA	1938	4	1958	
189 v3	Silvermines, Co. Tipperary	DNA	1934	12	1935	

Page No.	District	Scheme	Opened	Nurses	Closed	Longstanding Individual Nurses
199–365 v3	Skerries, Co. Dublin	DNA	1935	4	1966	Bridget O'Callaghan nee Clarke 1945–1966
157	Sligo District Nursing Association	DNA	1895	17	1960	Margaret Maloney 1937–1960
61–335 v3	Sneem, Co. Kerry	DNA	1928	15	1962	
217–18 v3	St Annes Hill & Inniscarra, Co. Cork	DNA	1937	12	1966	
7–8	St Laurence's Nurses' Home	DNA	1891	27	1955	
245–6 v3	St Margarets & Finglas, Co. Dublin	DNA	1940	3	1958	
325	St Marnocks, Malahide & Yellow Walls, Co. Dublin	DNA	1900	2	1904	
1–4	St Patrick's Nurses' Home	DNA	1867	49	1966	
349 v2	Stamullen, Co. Meath	WNHA	1911	6	1924	
45 v3	Stewardstown, Co. Tyrone	DNA	1925	1	1929	
121 v3	Stillorgan, Newtown Park, Deans Grange & Kill'o'the Grange, Co. Dublin	DNA	1932	4	1939	
73–5	Strabane, Co. Tyrone	DNA	1893	7	1932	Ellen Stanley 1912–1932
285–6 v3	Stradbally & Kilmacthomas, Co. Laois	DNA	1944	7	1958	
85–360 v3	Stradbally, Co. Laois	DNA	1930	12	1966	

Page No.	District	Scheme	Opened	Nurses	Closed	Longstanding Individual Nurses
191–2 v3	Stranorlor & Ballybofey, Co. Donegal	DNA	1934	8	1966	
271 v2	Sutton Home and Preventorium	WNHA	1906	2	1912	
559–61 v2	Swinford, Co.Mayo	LDS	1919	17	1967	Sarah Stewart 1939–1953
211	Swords & Donabate, Co. Dublin	DNA	1896	21	1966	
171–2 v3	Tallaght, Co. Dublin	DNA	1933	2	1956	
157–8 v2	Tandragee, Co. Armagh	WNHA	1909	5	1929	
249–50 v3	Taughboyne, Co. Donegal	DNA	1941	10	1967	
511 v2	Templemore & Dungloe, Co. Donegal	DNA	1917	1	1921	
223–4 v3	Termonfeckin, Co. Louth	DNA	1937	5	1956	
91	The Rosses, Co. Donegal	DNA	1893	2	1901	
97–100 v2	Thomastown, Co. Kilkenny	DNA	1908	17	1966	Leonora Ellison Doheny 1916–1935
223 v2	Thurles, Co. Tipperary	WNHA	1909	1	1911	
101 v3	Tinahealy, Co. Wicklow	DNA	1931	1	1935	
109–11 v2	Tipperary, Co. Tipperary	WNHA	1908	7	1955	Mary Angela Murphy 1919–1954
135 v3	Tourmakeady, Co. Mayo	LDS	1932	2	1935	
79–81 v2	Tralee, Co. Kerry	DNA	1908	14	1958	

Page No.	District	Scheme	Opened	Nurses	Closed	Longstanding Individual Nurses
25–308 v3	Tramore, Co. Waterford	DNA	1920	5	1966	
175–8 v2	Trim, Co. Meath	WNHA	1909	6	1967	Kathleen O'Grady 1911–1928; Florence Gilmartin 1929–1947
235–6 v3	Tullamore, Co. Offaly	DNA	1939	5	1966	Winifred Corr 1949–1966
91 v2	Tullamore, King's County (Now Co. Louth)	DNA	1908	1	1913	
157–381 v3	Tully & Spiddal, Co. Donegal	LDS	1933	10	1967	
421	Valentia Village Hospital, Co. Kerry	DNA	1872	2	1917	
169–71 v2	Valentia Village Hospital, Co. Kerry (Part 2)	DNA	1909	26	1967	
343 v3	Walkinstown, Co. Dublin	DNA	1958	3	1967	
397 v2	Warringstown, Co. Down	WNHA	1913	1	1915	
337–41	Waterford, Co. Waterford	DNA	1900	45	1966	Angela Sheedy 1937–1963
589–90 v2	Waterville, Co. Kerry	DNA	1919	4	1932	
205–8 v2	Westport, Co. Mayo	DNA	1909	10	1967	Ellen Joyce 1940–1967
37–8	Whitehouse; Whiteabbey; Greencastle, Co. Antrim	DNA	1892	7	1929	Emily Maude Halliday 1902–37
299–300 v3	Wicklow, Co. Wicklow	DNA	1950	3	1966	
105–404 v3	Youghal, Co. Cork	DNA	1931	9	192??	Mrs McGonigalnee Trainor 1942–66

Superintendents and Inspectors of the Queen's Institute of District Nursing in Ireland

SUPERINTENDENTS and INSPECTORS – 1890–1968	
1890–1899	Miss Mary Lucy Eliza Dunn
1899–1912	Miss Mary Lamont
1912–1928	Miss Annie Michie (Inspectors: Miss Mooney; Miss Cross)
1916	Miss Chisholm (acting in Miss Annie Michie's absence)
1928–1951	Miss Elizabeth Colburn (Inspectors: Miss Kavanagh; Miss Crothers; Miss Dowdy; Miss Fitzgerald; Miss Burke; Miss Aylward; Miss Kenny)
1951–1960	Miss F H Aylward (Inspector: Miss Burke)
1960–1968	Miss Mary Quain (Inspectors: Miss W. Burke; Miss M. Delaney)
1968	Queen's Institute of District Nursing ceased training in Ireland. Miss M Delaney, former Inspector of Queen's Institute of District Nursing, became Supervisor/Inspector with Lady Dudley's Scheme until it ceased operations in 1974.